Out Of Uniform And Into Trouble... Again

Carol D. DeYoung, RN, MS
*Margene Tower, RN, MS
Jody Glittenberg, RN, PhD, FAAN

First Edition Contributors

Phyllis Old Dog Cross Pearson - RN, MS

N. Jean Bauman, RN, MS

F. Jane Lockwood, RN, MS (deceased)

Virginia S. Paulson (deceased)

*This book was written by Margene Tower in her private capacity. No official support or endorsement by Indian Health Service is intended or should be inferred.

First Edition Copyright © 1971

Second Edition—Copyright © 1983, by SLACK Incorporated,
6900 Grove Road, Thorofare, New Jersey.
ISBN No. 0-913590-98-3
Library of Congress Catalog Card Number 12-62400

This Book Is
Dedicated to the Memory of

Virginia Belle Smith Paulson

1963-1980 - Executive Director, Colorado Nurses Association, Born: December 27, 1918, Died: August 9, 1982. Our first edition co-author, revered non-nurse leader of nurses, mentor, risk taker, and cherished friend.

Foreword
to the First Edition

Philosophy of life—
I'd pick more daisies

"If I had my life to live over, I'd try to make more mistakes next time. I would relax. I would limber up. I would be sillier than I have been this trip. I know of very few things I would take seriously. I would be crazier. I would be less hygienic. I would climb more mountains, swim more rivers and watch more sunsets. I would burn more gasoline. I would eat more ice cream and less beans. I would have more actual troubles and fewer imaginary ones. You see, I am one of those people who lives prophylactically and sensibly and sanely, hour after hour, day after day. Oh, I have had my moments, and, if I had it to do over again, I'd have more of them. In fact, I'd try to have nothing else. Just moments, one after another, instead of living so many years ahead each day. I have been one of those people who never go anywhere without a thermometer, a hot-water bottle, a gargle, a raincoat and a parachute. If I had it to do over again, I would go places and do things and travel lighter than I have. If I had my life to live over, I would start barefooted earlier in the spring and stay that way later in the fall. I would play hooky more. I wouldn't make such good grades except by accident. I would ride on more merry-go-rounds. I'd pick more daisies."

Anonymous

In the foreword of the first edition of *Out of Uniform and Into Trouble* we used this anonymous philosophy of life that we felt expressed the ideas we hoped you would find in the book. Since the book remains basically unchanged, the philosophy still fits and perhaps more so now than twelve years ago. If we intended to do any provoking, and we did, it was to provoke the entire mental health establishment to take itself less seriously, and if they had the chance, to do it better next time; in short, to pick more daisies. In view of what has occurred with mental health centers in the '70's and '80's, which we will address in the introductory chapter, you might find that eating ice cream and picking daisies should have been the priority.

Preface

In the first edition of *Out of Uniform and Into Trouble* the Task Force, a gang of seven, set forth to find out how other disciplines in mental health viewed nurses. Some opinions were cherishable and others less so. Nonetheless, as true researchers and plain honest folk we wrote openly, and sometimes humorously, all the good and bad and the brave and the cowardly. Through the subsequent years, as the Task Force went on to other things, several of us were often asked where people could get copies of the book, when would new editions be published; would we write again. The first edition, published by C. V. MOSBY, showed a funny cover with a zipper, symbolic of the move out of the traditional uniform. The title and cover were unusual for nursing, to say the least. The book was chosen by both Medical-Surgical Nursing reviewers and Psychiatric Nursing reviewers as 1972 American Journal of Nursing Book of the Year. Congresswoman, Shirley Chisholm, then running for President of the United States, said to a crowd of National Organization for Women supporters, "It's a book all women must read." The Task Force, now three, hopes that this second edition will be read by men as well as women and nurses in all fields of practice.

The original study which we present to you in its unadulterated format represented a survey of our then peers and co-workers. We knew that the role of the nurse was intertwined with that of other team members. We were increasingly aware that the role of the nurse was limited by the perceptions of other disciplines as well as nurses' perceptions of themselves.

The design of the original study was simple and consisted of inviting members of the same discipline from a variety of Colorado settings to address themselves to an open-ended questionnaire (see Appendix). The first hour of discussion was carried out exclusively by the invited group. Following this, members of the panel and Task Force engaged in dialogue. Our purpose in surveying other disciplines was in no way intended to have them define the nursing role, but rather to assess reality in terms of attitudes and opinions of other members of the mental health team. The disciplines interviewed were psychiatric technicians, social workers, psychiatrists and psychologists. Two panels of nurses were interviewed—those involved in clinical practice and those in administration and education. Curiosity further led us to interview an interdisciplinary panel. The data, as they emerged from the tape-recorded discussions, raised many critical issues that were relevant to all nurses. The relevance was validated by our own personal experiences as well as those of others and added to our data.

In this updated version, the original study remains intact. We did, however, do an informal survey of some of the original panel members and asked them to reread the first book and to comment about what they felt was the same and what had changed. We also used our literary license to ask some of our colleagues to read the first *Out of Uniform* and react to it essentially in the same way. It is from this information and the exchanges between the new Gang of Three that the new chapters of the book come.

The original panel participants whose titles appear as they were at the time of our study follows:

Lois Badger, *Psychiatric Technician, Fort Logan Mental Health Center, Denver, Colorado*

James T. Barter, *M.D., Staff Psychiatrist and Assistant Professor, Colorado Psychiatric Hospital and University of Colorado Medical Center, Denver, Colorado*

Ethel Bonn, *M.D., Director, Fort Logan Mental Health Center, Denver, Colorado*

Arlo Campbell, *Licensed Psychiatric Technician, Colorado State Hospital, Pueblo, Colorado*

Dorothy DiNero, *R.N., Colorado State Hospital, Pueblo, Colorado*

Jack Doose, *Licensed Psychiatric Technician, Colorado State Hospital, Pueblo, Colorado*

Evelyn Gaskill, *M.S.W., Arapahoe Comprehensive Mental Health Center, Englewood, Colorado*

Ernest L. Hall, *R.N., M.S., Assistant Professor of Psychiatric Nursing, University Of Colorado School of Nursing, Denver, Colorado*

Irene Hasche, *M.S.W., Psychiatric Social Worker, Colorado Psychiatric Hospital, Denver, Colorado*

Iris Holtje, *M.S.W., Emergency Psychiatric Services, University of Colorado Medical Center, Denver, Colorado*

Helen Huber, *RN., M.S., Chief of Nursing Service, Fort Logan Mental Health Center, Denver, Colorado*

Carol K. James, *RN., M.S., Nursing Service Director, Tri-County District Health Department, Englewood, Colorado*

Paul Jarvis, *Ph.D., Chief, Adult Psychiatry Division A, Fort Logan Mental Health Center, Denver, Colorado*

Art Jones, *Psychiatric Social Worker, Colorado State Hospital, Pueblo, Colorado*

Lennyce Kintner, *R.N., Director of Nursing, Bethesda Psychiatric Hospital, Denver, Colorado; former Task Force Member*

Gregorio Kort, *M.D., Director, Southern Division, Colorado State Hospital, Pueblo, Colorado*

Therese LaLancette, *R.N., M.P.H., Mental Health Nurse Consultant, U.S.P.H.S., N.I.M.H.; former Task Force Member*

Barbara Lee, *R.N., M.S., Colorado Psychiatric Hospital, Denver, Colorado*

Madeleine Leininger, *R.N., Ph.D., Director, Nurse-Scientist Program, University of Colorado School of Nursing, Denver, Colorado*

Dolores Leone, *R.N., M.S., Commnity Mental Health Center, Denver General Hospital, Denver, Colorado*

Pavel Machotka, *Ph.D., Colorado Psychiatric Hospital, Denver, Colorado*

Patricia Milich, *R.N., M.S., Director of Nursing, Colorado State Hospital, Pueblo, Colorado; former Task Force Member*

Charles E. Meredith, *M.D., Superintendent, Colorado State Hospital, Pueblo, Colorado*

Anabele Miller, *Psychiatric Technician, Colorado State Hospital, Pueblo, Colorado*

Dolores Milligan, *L.P.N., Community Mental Health Center, Denver General Hospital, Denver, Colorado*

Charles Oppegard, *M.D., Director, Bethesda Hospital, Denver, Colorado*

Seymour Opochinsky, *Ph.D., Denver University School of Psychology, Denver, Colorado*

Janet Palmer, *M.D., Community Mental Health Center, Denver General Hospital, Denver, Colorado*

Elizabeth Rose, *Psychiatric Technician, Colorado State Hospital, Pueblo, Colorado*

Nancy D. Sanford, *R.N., M.S., Instructor, St. Luke's Hospital School of Nursing, Denver, Colorado*

James Selkin, *Ph.D., Psychologist, Community Mental Health Center, Denver General Hospital, Denver, Colorado*

Vi Siewert, *Licensed Psychiatric Technician (now Mental Health Worker), Fort Logan Mental Health Center, Denver, Colorado*

Ed Van Natta, *M.S.W., Adams County Mental Health Center, Adams City, Colorado*

Henry Walzer, *M.S.W., Mental Health Center of Boulder County, Boulder, Colorado*

Richard Washburn, *Ph.D., Psychologist, Denver General Hospital, Denver, Colorado*

Georgia Westervelt, *M.S.W., Community Mental Health Center, Denver General Hospital, Denver, Colorado*

H. G. Whittington, *M.D., Director, Division of Psychiatry, Division of Health and Hospitals, Denver, Colorado*

Harl Young, *Ph.D., Colorado State Department of Institutions, Denver, Colorado*

Rothlyn Zahourek, *R.N., M.S., Community Mental Health Center, Denver General Hospital, Denver, Colorado*

We also wish to thank and acknowledge those people whose ideas are reflected in the 1983 book:

Karen Babich, *R.N., Ph.D., M.S., Western Interstate Commission of Higher Education, Boulder, Colorado*

Belle Burnsed, *R.N., M.S., Bethesda Mental Health Center, Denver, Colorado*

Jean Busherhoff, *R.N., Ph.D., Private Practice, Denver, Colorado*

Jeanette Chamberlain, *R.N., Ed.D., F.A.A.N., National Institute of Mental Health, Washington, D.C.*

Ann Cross, *R.N., B.S., Psychiatric Unit, St. Anthony's Hospital, Denver, Colorado*

Alice, Demi, *R.N., D.N.Sc., Georgia Medical College, Augusta, Georgia*

Gary Fletcher, *M.D., Private Psychiatrist, Denver, Colorado*

Jean Foland, *R.N., B.S., St. Anthony's Central Hospital, Denver, Colorado*

Dorothy Gregg, *R.N., M.S., F.A.A.N., University of Colorado School of Nursing, Denver, Colorado*

Leon Krier, *M.A., Psychiatric Unit, St. Anthony's Hospital, Denver, Colorado*

Madeleine Leininger, *R.N., Ph.D., F.A.A.N., Wayne State University, Detroit, Michigan*

Dolores Leone, *R.N., M.S., Bethesda Mental Health Center, Denver, Colorado*

Allan Levy, *M.D., Private Psychiatrist, Denver, Colorado*

Bern McCracken, *Ed.D., Clinical Psychologist, Private Practice, Denver, Colorado*

Don Moore, *M.A., Division of Mental Health Programs, Montana Department of Institutions, Helena, Montana*

Betty Mitsunaga, *R.N., Ph.D., F.A.A.N., University of Colorado School of Nursing, Denver, Colorado*

Gordon Neligh, *M.D., Area Mental Health Program, Indian Health Service, Billings, Montana*

Harriet Palmer-Willis, *R.N., M.S., Colorado Department of Health, Denver, Colorado*

Out of Uniform & Into Trouble . . . Again

William F. Rehg, *M.D., Private Psychiatrist, Denver, Colorado*

Carol Robbins, *R.N., B.S., Psychiatric Unit, St. Anthony's Central Hospital, Denver, Colorado*

Patricia M. Thomas, *R.N., M.S., Geriatric Nurse Consultant, Aurora, Colorado*

Patricia Uris, *R.N., M.S., Western Interstate Commission of Higher Education for Nursing, Boulder, Colorado*

Joe Vollmer, *M.S.W., Psychiatric Unit, St. Anthony's Hospital, Denver, Colorado*

Fran Walker, *Ph.D., Director of Human Resources Development Colorado Division of Mental Health, Denver, Colorado*

Nancy Wilson, *R.N., M.S., Director of Evaluation Services, Colorado Division of Mental Health, Denver, Colorado*

Rothlyn Zahourek, *R.N., M.S., Private Practice and Alcoholism Program Consultant, New York/ New Jersey*

Special thanks to numerous psychiatric nurses at the ANA Psychiatric Nursing Conference Group - ANA Biennial Convention, July 1, 1982; Psychiatric Nursing Conference, San Francisco, California, April, 1982; and a special recognition for the history makers at the Century Celebration; Psychiatric Nursing in Historical Perspectives, sponsored by Journal of Psychosocial Nursing and Mental Health Services and Charles B. Slack, Inc.

Invaluable insight was gained from the Generation Panel Luncheon at the Century Celebration. Speakers at the Luncheon included:

Ann W. Burgess, *R.N., D.N.Sc., F.A.A.N.*

Esther Garrison, *R.N., D.N.Sc., L.L.D., F.A.A.N. (hon.)*

June Mellow, *R.N. Ed.D.*

Dorothy Mereness, *R.N., Ed.D.*

Hildegard Peplau, *R.N., Ed.D., F.A.A.N.*

Shirley A. Smoyak, *R.N., Ph.D., F.A.A.N.*

Dorris Stewart, *R.N., M.S.*

Contents

PART ONE
An Update

Chapter One

A DECADE OF CHANGE

The decade following the first edition of *Out of Uniform and Into Trouble* was remarkable. The end to the fighting in Vietnam left scars that may never heal and questions that may never be answered as to why and how as a nation we engaged in such a war. Children recently carrying flowers were now impatiently resisting a war of unknown cause. As they were felled by National Guard bullets at Kent State, a nation finally rose in horror to say "No More!" Still we are yet concerned and pained by the returned veteran who was scorned and forgotten.

The troubled decade had moments of greatness as a President renewed alliances and walked along the Great Wall of China only to be brought down in disgrace by a self-serving cover-up. Expletives deleted and eighteen minutes of silence became symbolic of the national agony captured in one word . . . Watergate. A nation whose very self-image had nearly been destroyed found renewed strength when Congress made the system work. Out of the confusion came an extraordinary longing for simplicity and honesty and . . . healing.

It was a time when a peanut farmer from Georgia, who was also a nuclear physicist, was elected President. He, a graduate of Annapolis, spoke with humility and welcomed an impressive March of the Poor to the Capitol in Washington, D.C. Yet, he could not gather a united constituency for re-election as a tense nation awaited release of fifty-one American hostages captured in Iran.

The ice person cometh

His replacement in the White House, a former movie star and governor of a populous state, took over the leadership of the nation. His corporate image makers painted a picture of success even as world inflation skyrocketed and our national economy plunged toward a depression with unprecedented unemployment.

Tax cuts, tax increases, massive cuts in social programs with massive increases in military spending confused every one except the Office of Management and Budget Director. It has become clear since then that only our nation's priorities have changed and not the size or expansion of the national budget. Afternoon soap operas offer escapes from the increasing horrors reported to us on early morning, noon, early nightly and late nightly news. The Age of Causes has been replaced with the Age of Isms, i.e. Feminism, Sexism, Ageism. Federal fiscal priorities reflect the new elitism with social concern at the bottom of the heap. Weapons development received almost unlimited monies while social sciences research received the equivalent of the Proxmire Golden Fleece Award.

Women have not fared well in this decade. There has been a growing backlash from the late '60's and early '70's when Gloria Steinem, Shirley Chisholm, and Betty Friedan dominated the Women's Movement. The backlash that developed was lead by Phyllis Schlafly and her "total women," Stepford wives . . . wearing the same smiles and uniformly dressed. The most eloquent evidence that women have not fared well in this decade was the failure of the Equal Rights Amendment to win passage in 1982. The ERA's defeat meant that this society could not deal with a phrase that simply said— there shall be no discrimination under the law on the basis of sex. What is at stake for society in keeping over half of its population in an inequitable position under the law? A major reason may be found in the marketplace, for it would cost industry and government billions of dollars to pay women at a comparable rate with men. Therefore it seems to us inequality not equality makes the world go round.

Nonetheless, where do we look for answers? We believe the Women's Movement lost its focus by trying to address a multiplicity of ideas and issues. The issues of abortion, gay rights and the draft, to name a few, were divisive and became red herrings which were used to draw us off the path and away from the fundamental issue . . . a simple one of prohibiting discrimination on the basis of sex according to the Constitution. We would be remiss, though, if we didn't say that something was learned. What was learned is that the name of the tune is economics. Now the critical need is to use the legislative process and not to repeat the mistakes that led to the defeat of ERA.

The issues we have just addressed all have had an impact on nursing. So, how has mental health nursing fared in this decade? Some of the predictions made in the first edition have come true, i.e., there has been movement of mental health professionals including nursing into private practice; mental health centers have become mental illness centers as increasing numbers of people with alcoholism, drug addiction, criminal behavior and the deinstitutionalization of the chronically mentally ill has swelled caseloads.

We had hoped in 1971 that the number of psychiatric nurses in mental health centers would increase. In fact we found that the number of nurses in Colorado Mental Health Centers in 1981, by percentage, was identical to the numbers in 1969.[1] Instead of increases in staffing of mental health centers we found decreases. More than one clinician contacted said, "Mental health centers are dead." They also said, "Nurses are moving into private practice and other community settings;—not that there were ever that many nurses

---

[1] Colorado Division of Mental Health Report, 1981.

in mental health centers in the first place, you understand." Another trend, nurses (many more than just psychiatric nurses) have gone out of uniform in the last decade. For instance, a nursing cap is seldom seen these days. Identity and status come more in the form of plastic color-coded I.D. cards that look very much like a driver's license or a security guard badge. In 1971 nurses wanted a more prominent role as therapists in mental health centers. They didn't get it. In the 1970's the vast majority of the population and our professional colleagues did not "buy" the nurse as an addition to the Holy Trinity or Grand Triumverate of psychiatrists, psychologists and social workers. We discussed many of the reasons this might be true in the first edition. Unfortunately we find that the concept of the marginal man still holds true, i.e., if a discipline is not part of the original group they are doomed to forever remain on the fringes.

Ask not for whom the bell tolls

Power as an issue was discussed in the first edition at some length. We hoped that power would give way to sharing for the common good. That common good was to see that optimal health care was available. That hope seems now, at best, naive. There is no notion of sharing the turf these days, as rights to practice are won only in the courts. It is a paradox that when nurses push for their rights as professionals and for the rights of patients to receive the best quality of care, they are accused of being self-serving and aggressive, and when nurses are compromising, passive, or compassionate, they are accused by the Women's Movement of representing all the worst characteristics of women. What we see occurring as nurses try to assert some power is a cycle of action . . . inaction . . . reaction regarding issues in which nursing has a vital interest. A good example of this is the Health Care Technicians' role which was proposed by Denver Health and Hospitals in Colorado. The Health Care Technician was to provide a cheap source of labor to do everything from taking patients' histories, doing preliminary testing on all psychiatric patients, providing oral and intramuscular medication, starting IVs to educating patients about the side effects of drugs, to performing independent home nursing care for noncritical patients. Yes, dear reader, that's correct . . . you read it right, the Health Care Technician was to do all those things with no more than the requirement that they be able to read and write.[2]

It seems unbelievable that such a proposal could win official approval, but it did. Then, you may ask, what happened? Nurses across the country were alarmed by the action of the Denver Personnel System and said so loudly, and in print, and at least in Colorado, in press conferences and in testimony at city council meetings. Then, a group of nurses in Colorado worked hard to get resolutions passed in the nursing and public health professional orga-

---

[2] Job Description Health Care Technician I–IV. Denver Health and Hospital Career Service Authority, June 1, 1980.

nizations opposing the use of Health Care Technicians. These organized, insightful nurses were concerned with protecting the health and safety of the citizens of Colorado. The nurse-sponsored resolutions, after much debate and political machinations, were passed.[3,4] But, we are sad to say, no follow-up of any consequence to date occurred from these state professional organizations. It would have made a great deal of sense to have discussed this critical health care issue at a national level, as these are the kinds of things nursing leaders are talking about when they fear for the survival of nursing. In an editorial[5] letter from nursing leader, Dr. Rozella Schlotfeldt, she stated, "I am concerned about what I see as mounting evidence that a genuine threat to nursing's continued progress or even survival exists . . ."[6] Her concern was based on the closure of some of the nation's finest private schools of nursing at Stanford, Cornell and the University of Chicago. Even more frightening, because it represents an open attack against nursing leadership and the naked exercise of power against nursing, is her chronicling of the firing of prominent nurses in education and nursing services. Dr. Schlotfeldt asked, "Is nursing consistently to be undermined by others whose power may be threatened?" The editor responds to state that nursing is in a vulnerable transition period and that we must make sure that those who stick their necks out don't get their throats cut.[7] We, the authors, add that if we don't pay attention, we may find ourselves going the way of the dinosaurs, i.e., into extinction to be rediscovered some day under heaps of Sunset Review documents, position descriptions for untrained health technicians, and applications for third party reimbursement which were returned stamped "disallowed." The day may come when professional nurse positions will be reclassified as Health Care Technician. Some nurse administrators will no doubt be found justifying this kind of action. They will use arguments such as military precedence ("The military services have used 'these' people for years") never having read books such as Aynes's book on Army Nursing where Aynes describes the horrors and dangers of the use of non-professional workers.[8] These nurse administrators will stand behind their physician bosses and forget their commitment to the highest level of patient care.

Ghost of seasons past

You might ask, where were we, the authors of this book, during the upheaval over the Equal Rights Amendment in the late '70's. We remained true to the colors we raised in the first edition of the book concerning the obvious

---

[3] Colorado Public Health Association Resolution Convention, June 1981.
[4] Colorado Nurses' Association Resolution, House of Delegates, April 1981.
[5] Scorr, T. Nursing Leaders: an Endangered Species. American Journal of Nursing, February 1982, p. 313.
[6] Ibid.
[7] Ibid.
[8] Aynes, E.A. From Nightingale to Eagle. Englewood Cliffs, N.J.: Prentice-Hall, Inc., 1973.

second-class citizenship of women and nurses by contributing all of the royalties from the first book to The Colorado Nurses' Association for political action on behalf of nursing. We also, through the Colorado Nurses' Association, supported and contributed monies to NURSE Incorporated for the Class Action Suit brought by Lemons, et al, against the Denver Health and Hospital System. That suit demanded equal pay for work of comparable worth and responsibility within the city-county government. ANA also monetarily supported this suit and passed a resolution in 1978 around this issue.[9] A federal court judge ruled against the suit on the basis of the overwhelming economic impact it would have. The suit went through the court system up to the Supreme Court which did not choose to hear the case. What does that tell you, dear reader? Economics is the name of the tune. Again and again, with the Equal Rights Amendment, in the priorities for government spending and in the attack against nursing there has been a distressing sense of powerlessness which we feel should be addressed. Nurses and women have not been powerless in terms of numbers, but in a lack of focus and unity and a failure to perceive the enemy (which includes ourselves). The authors have had the recurring nightmare that some day, when enough fragmentation has occurred, someone, the big "theys" in the sky, will demand an accounting of nursing's right to exist and we'll all stand there with blank looks on our faces stuttering and mumbling something about quality of patient care, and we'll lose. Then we'll be angry at the injustice of it all and shuffle off to dens to brood. The strange thing is, we still think, as we did twelve years ago, that quality of patient care is *exactly* "Where it's at." We must become far more effective in articulating and demonstrating that value to the public if the profession is to survive. It is insufficient and, we think, probably downright irritating to people to rave on about conceptual frameworks and nursing diagnosis in trying to explain the value of professional nurses. The outcomes are what count in this age of microdots and management by objectives; and *good outcomes are there*; they just haven't been effectively demonstrated to the public for all the reasons we have talked about in this chapter and in the subsequent chapters.

So it has been a frustrating decade, and, all things considered, the bottom line in this age of bottom lines is, what has changed? Not very much. So, read the next few chapters as they were written twelve years ago and laugh and weep and maybe go pick some daisies until you reach the last chapters when we perhaps will have regained some optimism.

---

[9] Nurse, Inc. A Case for Cooking. Denver, Colo.: 1980, pp. 166–167.

PART TWO
Nursing—as others see us

Chapter Two

ROBOTS OR REBELS— THE RATIONALE FOR A STUDY

Picture a fat guy and a skinny guy on a teeter-totter. The fat guy does all the work but still doesn't get off the ground except by his own strength. The skinny guy looks as if he's having all the fun and sitting on high. A crude analogy, but applicable to the feeling many nurses have about their positions in community mental health action. In order to shed some enlightenment upon this unbalanced situation, our Task Force investigated how the various players within community mental health centers viewed the position of the nurse on the team—the fat guy on a teeter-totter.

Earlier studies

Glittenberg in 1962 conducted a national survey of the nurse's role in outpatient psychiatric clinics (before the 1963 Community Mental Health Centers Act) and found that *fewer than ten percent* of the facilities even included a nurse on the professional team. In addition, the Glittenberg survey identified a wide diversity of functions the nurse in these few settings perceived herself performing. To complicate the situation further, clinics employed nurses with academic backgrounds varying from the two-year associate degree programs through doctoral preparation, and all had the identical title of "nurse." A dilemma occurred among the nurses with master's and doctorate degrees who believed they were "boxed in." They were prepared academically to function more broadly, but their skills were not being recognized by other disciplines. Because of this frustration, employment was often sought elsewhere.

That 1962 survey noted that nurses were performing a wide variety of functions. More than fifty percent were participating in initial interviews as co-therapists, making home visits, and were functioning in liaison capacities. Academic backgrounds were not necessarily related to the type of functions nurses were performing.[1] Sixty-one percent of the nurses were employed part time, with diploma graduates comprising forty-two percent of the respondents. The full-time nurses assisted more with physical therapies, such as dispensing drugs, and served more frequently as co-therapist directly to the patient. The part-time nurses were making more home visits and initial interview activities. A higher percentage of diploma graduates than nurses with a master's degree were performing clerical duties. It was obvious that the

---

[1] Glittenberg, J. A.: The role of the nurse in outpatient psychiatric clinics, The American Journal of Orthopsychiatry **39**:1, July 1963.

nurses with master's and doctorates could perform more direct therapy functions.

The unrelatedness of academic training to functions performed suggested that the nurse tended to operate as a broad generalist depending upon the unique demands of the clinic in which she was employed. Trouble and discontent seemed to stem more from the highly educated nurse who wanted recognition of her abilities and more opportunity to perform in a colleague relationship.[2]

A survey done in 1969 by Reres concluded that the registered nurse was identified as a psychiatric nurse in half the clinics, and in one-fourth she was seen as a public health nurse.[3]

The findings of still another study conducted at Maimonides Medical Center from 1963 to 1968, were published in *The Roles of Psychiatric Nurses in Community Mental Health Practice: A Giant Step*. This study notes that most psychiatric nurse clinicians believed they had little or no chance of being viewed by members of the other disciplines as peers or colleagues, but the members of the project that conducted this study found that each nurse had to justify herself in terms of her own skill and competence as did all other members of the staff of the center.[4] It was concluded that a dialogue should be maintained continuously between the nurse clinicians and the other disciplines, focusing specifically on roles, because these roles were continually changing. In this study it was noted that the organizational structure of the clinic delimited the roles of staff members. Therefore, if nurses were to effect changes in these structures, they would have to learn the rules of the game and become agents of change within their own settings.[5]

The director of Maimonides Medical Center, Dr. Montague Ullman, believed that prepared psychiatric nurses are an untapped source of able personnel. From his relationship with psychiatric nurses, he concluded they were prepared to participate as peer professionals rather than in ancillary or supporting roles.[6] These roles that prepared nurses could perform were differentiated by the nurses in the project as: (1) the generic clinician role shared with other members of the staff, (2) the legally defined role on hospital units, (3) providing informal aspects of hospital living for patients, and (4) ward coordination, matching patient needs with availability of staff and programs in the hospitalization units. It was apparent that the nurse was the team

---

[2] *Ibid*, p. 117.
[3] Reres, M. E.: A survey of the nurse's role in psychiatric outpatient clinics in America, Community Mental Health Journal **5**(5): 385, Oct. 1969.
[4] Stokes, G. A., Williams, F. S., Davidites, R. M., Bulbulyan, A., and Ullman, M.: The roles of psychiatric nurses in community mental health practice: a giant step, New York, 1969, Faculty Press, Inc., pp. 57–58.
[5] *Ibid*, p. 135.
[6] *Ibid*, p. 3.

member who displayed the greatest sensitivity to the overall patient population both on an informal level and in structured programs.[7]

We had surveyed our own positions as we, too, had experienced being in hot water on many occasions when we ventured beyond the narrow confines of the traditional nursing role and dared to give an opinion. Our professional status was often challenged; co-workers tested our abilities. One remark made by a social worker to one of the authors was, "You're like Jackie Robinson making the Big League." Another team member stated, "I didn't know you were a nurse! I like you, but I never liked nurses!"

Nursing is not unique in this struggle for identity. Writings appear continually in the journals about the social worker, psychologist, and psychiatrist's similar struggles. Each seems to be concerned with many of the issues we have faced in this book.[8,9]

All three of these early studies were conducted by nurses about their role. All revealed discontent among the "fat guys" and urged dialogues with other disciplines to seek clarification of the reasons for the exclusion of the nurse clinician or the rationale for inhibiting roles and the lack of colleague status with other team members. Following the recommendations of these studies, an interdisciplinary inquiry became the basis for our study. Nurses too frequently have been identified as passive followers. Critics reading this book may question if this passive pattern is again being repeated by questioning other disciplines about the nurse's role. No! Defining this role was viewed as an interactional process with other disciplines. Therefore, by reflecting on this interdisciplinary appraisal, nurses will have more data upon which to accept or to change the role they are carving out within community mental health centers. Other disciplines, too, may reassess their roles in these centers as they gain more awareness of the "fat guy" and where he wants to go.

During the past decade many changes have occurred in the delivery of mental health care in our society. Community psychiatry is in the fore. Decentralization of the century-old system of isolation from the community of the deviates identified as mentally ill has had an impact upon the professions delivering this care. Even the communities needed to develop a different frame of reference for the person labeled mentally ill. Crisis intervention, walk-in clinics, short-term hospitalization, and long-term follow-up have all become treatment modalities.

The now-famous message to Congress by the late President John F. Kennedy in 1963 on mental health and mental retardation ushered in a new era in which comprehensive mental health centers were to become the treatment

---

[7] *Ibid*, p. 134.

[8] Yolles, S. F.: The role of the psychologist in comprehensive community mental health center, American Psychologist, Jan. 1966, p. 40.

[9] Freeman, H. E., and Gertner, R. S.: The changing posture of the mental health consortium, American Journal of Orthopsychiatry **39**(1): 116, Jan. 1969.

centers for individuals within the community. Each center was to be designed specifically with the flexibility required to meet the needs of the communities. No single staffing pattern was proposed, but each center was to provide six basic services for the community: twenty-four hour inpatient treatment, partial hospitalization, outpatient services, emergency service, consultation, and research. It was estimated in 1963 that by early 1980, 2,500 centers, each serving a population between 75,000 and 200,000, would be in operation.[10] These new treatment modalities made new alignment of functional roles necessary, and this wasn't easy. Consequently, role confusion has resulted. New lines of communication between the team members have resulted. Old organizational structures have bent or crumbled. The greatest impact of these role changes is felt in the work situation where roles are extended, blurred, and fused. Risk-taking has become a common daily occurrence. Only those with iron guts can withstand the continual testing. "I'll cry tomorrow" became the motto of one group struggling for identity. How a group of professional mental health workers can survive and evolve into a new species could be viewed as a goal, but is beyond the rationale for this study. No one professional group can solve successfully the complexity of problems rising from this change.

Looking at the system

Social system theory identifies a system as being stable when each member knows where he belongs within that system. In our society, mental health care is only one part of a much larger health care institution. Technological and scientific advances in the last few decades have radically altered the structure of health care institutions. Furthermore, more demands have been placed upon medical services by the very fact of the population explosion and a gigantic increase in urbanization. To meet these demands, a vast network of interdependent organizations similar to a can of worms has developed. The complexity of these organizations has imposed specialization of functions, and specialization is accompanied by a fragmentation of delivery of services and a narrowing of focus.[11]

The health institutions only mirror the changes that are occurring on yet a broader basis, that of our total culture. Spindler has concluded that a new value system is emerging within our society that is characterized by social adaptability, relativism, and sensitivity to the opinions of others. The evidence of this is seen in the many movements of our day, such as the hippie, peace, and feminist movements. Traditional roles are being challenged in all fields[12] including military, religion, and law.

---

[10] Dorsett, C.: New directions in mental health facilities, The American Institute of Architects, Nov. 1964, p. 4.
[11] Smith, L. M.: The system—barriers to quality nursing. In Folta, J. R., and Deck, E. S., editors: A sociological framework for patient care, New York, 1966, John Wiley & Sons, Inc., p. 53.
[12] Spindler, G. D.: Group values—traditional and emergent. In Carter, H. J., editor: Intellectual foundations of American education, New York, 1965, Pitman Publishing Corp., p. 361.

Who is the patient?

The role of the patient also needs to be discussed in the rationale for this study. Talcott Parsons points out that the role of the patient in a health care system is defined culturally. It is the cultural system that defines whose behavior is deviant and whether it should be treated as an illness or by some other means of societal control. The hospital also has a unique cultural role in that it determines what kind of a deviant is to be treated there and how the rest of society is expected to act toward him. Hospitalization serves the function of socializing both the patient and the community to their proper response roles.[13]

This socialization process has changed considerably in the last two or three decades in psychiatry. Hospitalization of the mentally ill was frequently a lifetime process. Within the confines of custodial care, the patient was identified clearly in his role, and the community could clearly adjust to his absences. Now, however, with open-door and short-term therapy, who can separate the roles of patient and healthy citizen! It must be a disconcerting dilemma to those who long for the traditionally tight, defined roles. Others are willing to predict that this state of change is only temporary—the extreme swing of the proverbial pendulum will again stabilize and traditional roles will again emerge.

However, not all agree that the roles have changed this much. For instance, Albee does not see that there have been any real changes. "There is nothing on the inside [community mental health center] except the same old performers going through the same old routines."[14] Within a center, it becomes apparent that status is maintained by monopolizing certain functions, and these functions are further supported by explicit norms of certification, such as psychiatrist or registered nurse.[15] The symbol of status in psychiatry still is that of being an individual therapist. As functions and goals within a center have changed, most professionals are experiencing some identity crisis because of the emphasis on commonality and de-emphasis on discipline.[16]

Out of uniform

The rationale for this study is based on the facts that society is undergoing major changes, that health systems are straining to adapt, and accordingly, participants within the health professions are experiencing role change. This change hurts some more than others. Close observers of this metamorphosis may witness a phenomenon known as role distance. This is a term used by

[13] Parsons, T.: On becoming a patient. In Folta, J. R., and Deck, E. S., editors: A sociological framework for patient care, New York, 1966, John Wiley & Sons, Inc., p. 248.
[14] Albee, G. W.: No magic here, Contemporary Psychology, vol. 10, Sept. 1965, p. 497.
[15] Freeman and Gertner, *op cit*, p. 121.
[16] Stokes, *op cit*, p. 62.

sociologists to describe the process by which persons step out of a role to signal to others that they are not really to be identified with the part: "I'm not really a nurse—I just play like I am." However, neither the nurses on the Task Force nor the nurse clinicians in this study are denying their generic identification, but rather are recognizing the obligations of a new colleague role and are ready to assume the responsibilities demanded. One way of signaling other disciplines to this role change is dress. Laying aside the white or blue uniform for street clothes in public health and psychiatric settings began over a decade ago. This change was more than mere convenience; it was also a sign of behavioral change. *Out of Uniform and Into Trouble* is more than a catchy subtitle; it describes a role change.

Role change is tough. With each new member added to the system, the roles of the other members are challenged. The socialization ritual identified in changing from one position in society to another is called *rite de passage*. Gertrude Stokes candidly refers to this ritual in *Giant Step*. Nurse clinicians were submitted to testing of their knowledge and skill as a right to occupy a position at the mental health center. The *rite de passage* serves an important function in preparing a person to occupy a position more securely, because both he and the other team members know his assets.[17]

What does this role change entail? A brief description of nursing history will serve to identify some of its cultural past, which continues to influence practitioners today, and its continuing impact on other disciplines as well.

Light the lamp—there's a long way yet to go

Historically, nursing has usually been practiced in a dependent relationship with the physician. Cave drawings indicate that prehistoric man had a system of caring for the sick among his tribe. As the society of man became more organized, certain duties were delegated to individuals within the tribe. Sickness in an individual or a tribe was closely related to the whims of powerful ruling spirits. Thus, the treatment of the sick began as spirit-chasing by men designated this role by their clan. These men became prominent in restoring the sick to states of wellness. Can one doubt, then, where the origin of this omnipotent mystique surrounding physicians arose? If one bothers to look closely at the caste of medicine men, one can see an assistant who is definitely an inferior class of practitioner applying the treatment prescribed by the medicine man. This inferior associate was often an old women of the tribe. No doubt, the original dyad of doctor-nurse, physician-assistant had its beginning in ancient history. Studying this established pattern of dominance-submission relationship reveals that this pattern continues to the present day, although in a modified form. In 1969, an American Nurses' Association survey

---

[17] Stokes, *op cit*, p. 198.

revealed that the greatest single response to the question of how nurses should operate was *to assist the physician*.[18] Few would argue that the physician holds the highest professional status in American society. A phenomenon has been noted in academic circles that only physicians retain the title "Dr." even in company of Ph.D.'s, some of whom are registered nurses who have more years of academic preparation.

Before Christianity care of the sick was neglected. The teachings of Christianity stress the need to love one's neighbor as oneself, and ministering to fellow man was a means of imitating the life of Christ. It was the Crusade Knights who erected hospitals and initiated nursing orders. Nursing has strong roots in religion and military institutions. No wonder it is so traditionally bound!

Until a century ago, nursing was an art learned in apprenticeship. This, indeed, was not different from other professions such as law, medicine, and teaching. However, it should be noted that in 1869, at a meeting of the American Medical Association, it was recommended that nursing education be placed under the control of the medical profession. It was proposed that every large hospital train nurses.[19] This recommendation did not pass, but the concept proposed continues to influence nursing to this day.

Although such early leaders in nursing as Isabel Hampton Robb urged that nursing education be maintained separately from service to hospitals, their voices had little influence for half a century. Nursing education was closely aligned with giving service to the hospitals. To hospital administrators this apprenticeship became one of the chief means of staffing the hospital. Hospital training schools flourished for over fifty years. A survey financed by the Rockefeller Foundation, known as the Golmark Report of 1922, cried out against the deficiencies in nursing education. The most significant conclusion was: schools of nursing could not meet both goals—that of caring for the sick and that of educating the nurse.[20]

Education for nursing in hospital training schools only began to decline after World War II when nurses were financially able to attend college with GI Bill benefits. Following Sputnik I, the whole nation became college hungry. The leadership and financial benefits that resulted from attaining a baccalaureate degree overshadowed the benefits graduates of diploma schools received, and these schools have begun to close their doors. Independent thinkers have been in the making, and college-prepared nurses are becoming discontent with their status on the health team.

A population boom, urbanization, scientific breakthroughs, technology,

---

[18] Nurses, nursing and the ANA, The American Journal of Nursing **70**(4):809, April 1970.
[19] Dolan, J: History of nursing, ed. 12, Philadelphia, 1968, W. B. Saunders Co., p. 218.
[20] *Ibid*, p. 323.

and third-party hospitalization insurance have put more demands on the health care system. The old dyad of doctor-nurse is out of date—the team has expanded to a small army. Nursing has had to meet the challenge of change.

Unrest among the ranks

Among the nursing profession itself, myriad problems exst. First, who has the right to the title R.N.? The associate degree or two-year graduate, the four- or five-year baccalaureate, or the many in-betweens? One state board nurse examination for all these levels confers the title of R.N. after the name (and each state designates its own "passing" score). How incredible to measure the learning of five years with that of two by means of the same examination. When can highly innovative scholars and clinicians finally reconcile that there are differences that should be measured and titled by different means. Surely, then, some of the confusion as to which "kind" of nurse's role we are defining would diminish.

Hopelessly outdated Nurse Practice Acts hem in the nurse, both from above and below. Innovative nursing often is curtailed by the stifling clause ". . . must be practiced under the supervision of a physician." On the other hand, an army of subprofessionals are directly responsible to the registered nurse, making her moves as free as those of the Old Woman in a Shoe!

The whole baseline for this inquiry into the role of the nurse is not complete until one considers the sexual identity of the vast majority of nurses. With the rise of the feminist movement, many of the issues expressed by activists of this movement are also applicable to nursing. The hierarchy of doctor over nurse will be questioned along the lines of male-female roles. It is *not* obviously natural, as some claim, that men should be dominant and women submissive. Shuffle, baby, shuffle! As women socialized in our society, we have been taught to be passive, dependent, and submissive. Even as children, our defenses were verbal, rarely physical. To be creative, other than child bearing, or intelligent, categorized a woman as a castrating female. To quote Lucy Komisar: "At the center of the feminist critique, is the recognition that women have been forced to accept an inferior role in society and that we have come to believe in our own inferiority. Women are taught to be passive, dependent, submissive, not to pursue careers but to be taken care of and protected."[21] Women, furthermore, have been brow-beaten into believing that if they become competitive like men, the home will fold and society crumble! A rigid society that forces individuals into molds because of race, religion, sex, or whatever, loses that individual's spontaneity and potential.

This, then, is the purpose of this book—that the potential of the nurse's role be fully developed rather than be subjected to stifling molds. The ra-

---

[21] Komisar, L.: The new feminism, Saturday Review, February 21, 1970, p. 28.

tionale for the study is best summarized, we think, not by contemporary social scientists, but by the ancient scholar, Aristotle:

> No one is able to attain the truth adequately, while on the other hand, we do not collectively fail, but everyone says something true about the nature of things, and while individually we contribute little or nothing to the truth, by the union of all a considerable amount is amassed.

Chapter Three

THE VIEW
FROM THE TOP —
OR PSYCHIATRISTS LET
THEIR HAIR DOWN

After the decision was made to interview representatives from various professional groups, plans had to be finalized regarding whom to contact from which professions. Because psychiatrists were at the top of the established hierarchy of the mental health professions and many were the administrative heads of institutions and centers, the Task Force felt that it was appropriate to hold the first interview with the psychiatrist-administrators of the largest mental health institutions in Colorado. This group of four psychiatrists, who represented the public-sector psychiatrist, were not only the heads of large medical-state bureaucracies but also were identified by the Task Force as leaders in their field.

It was recognized that the first group of psychiatrists were not a representative sample of Colorado psychiatrists, so it was decided to later invite a second group of psychiatrists, who hopefully, would represent a different philosophy or impression concerning the nurse's role in the comprehensive community mental health center. These psychiatrists were from the private sector. Alas, it was from this group that we had the poorest response. Only two of those invited came, and only one was truly representative of the private sector per se.

At first, we attempted to separate the responses of the two groups of psychiatrists into two reports. However, because of the similarity of the two interviews, it was decided to integrate the so-called public-sector group with the group from the private sector. Themes were identified and organized from the two interviews. (How exciting the discussion would have been had all six members been on the same panel.)

There was a total of six psychiatrists in the two groups. Three of the psychiatrists were women. The Task Force pondered among ourselves whether female physicians would be more supportive or more restrictive toward nurses and their role. As it turned out, one of the strongest supporters of the nurse was a woman, and one of the most restrictive of the group was a man.

In preparation for writing this book, the Task Force members discussed and analyzed the transcriptions from the two interviews. It was no surprise to find that the psychiatrists labeled as representatives of the public sector revealed themselves to be more liberal than those from the private sector.

As Goffman states, "Social settings establish the categories of persons likely to be encountered there."[1] In this chapter, we will deal with the social settings

---

[1] Goffman, E.: Stigma: notes on the management of spoiled identity, Englewood Cliffs, N.J., 1965, Prentice-Hall, Inc., p. 2.

of the mental hospital and the community mental health center. The persons encountered will be the psychiatrist, nurse, and patient. Goffman goes on further to describe the phenomenon of the communication system within a setting. "These routines of social intercourse in established settings allow us to deal with anticipated others without special attention or thought."[2]

The fact that the hospital and, even more significantly, the mental hospital are social settings has been well documented. Loeb pointed out that "The social structure of this hospital is very complicated. There is a professional status system which ranges from the physician at the top through social workers, psychologists and nurses to the lowly maintenance and kitchen help."[3]

Leifer has found that "The bureaucratization and technicalization of medical practice permit psychiatry to be practiced in an institutional setting and still retain a similarity to medicine."[4] He goes on further to describe the function of the psychiatrist administrator. "The mental hospital administrator autocratically rules a professional staff arranged in a strict hierarchy of authority."[5] His final point is that in this hierarchy the lower echelon is the one that supervises the patient group.

Why were the public sector psychiatrists we interviewed more liberal than the private sector psychiatrists? Several theories were offered by the Task Force but none could be validated. One concerned the fact that the two psychiatrists from the State Hospitals in Colorado were both accustomed to working with nurses in all phases of a community mental health program. Also, the State Hospitals in Colorado are not the traditional state hospital as it is generally perceived. Both are oriented toward providing a center for comprehensive community mental health care. These psychiatrists had more knowledge of what a nurse could do in the areas of day care, after care, consultation, planning, and evaluation. Some of the public psychiatrists who were younger and perhaps more liberal in their thinking about mental health were extremely restrictive and rigid in their perceptions of the nurse's role in community mental health. This inflexible view could probably be associated with their inexperience in working or associating with nurses in other than inpatient settings. Another theory was that the administrative psychiatrists were well established in their social settings; therefore, they could feel free to recognize the contributions of nurses who are lower in status. The psychiatrists who had less status in their own systems were in need of a more rigid system and were less tolerant of the upward mobility of lower status professionals.

In our analysis of these sessions several intense and heated discussions

---

[2] *Ibid.*

[3] Loeb, M. B.: Some dominant cultural themes in a psychiatric hospital. In Spitzer, S. P., and Denzin, N. K., editors: The mental patient; studies in the sociology of deviance, New York, 1968, McGraw-Hill Book Co., p. 306.

[4] Leifer, R.: In the name of mental health, New York, 1969, Science House, Inc., p. 73.

[5] *Ibid*, p. 139.

ensued, and ideas were tested on colleagues and peers. Themes from the interviews with psychiatrists were identified and researched. These themes included doctor-nurse relationships, the traditional nurse, the woman-nurse, the nurse in the community mental health center, and nursing education. There will be some questions posed and some hypotheses offered based on the ideas and opinions of the psychiatrists as presented to the Task Force.

Nurse-doctor relationships—or keeping the seat warm

One of the most intriguing relationships that occurs among the mental health professionals is that unique bond between the nurse and the doctor. This relationship has been romanticized by literature, television, and movies. Perhaps the epitome of this version is that of Rex Morgan, M.D. and his nurse June. June is depicted as ever-faithful, devoted, dependent, and helpful. There is always a hint of a possible romance that is never fulfilled. The relationship remains pure and professional and June remains virginal in her omnipresent white uniform. We have taken an informal survey among nurse colleagues, and there is not one nurse to be found who likes June or regards her as a role model for nurses. This relationship is referred to in nursing circles as the handmaiden relationship and it is seen as being perpetuated by doctors and nurses alike.

The military-religious background of nursing resulted in an end product who behaved both like a nun and a first sergeant. Nurses were encouraged both by their training and the system to develop a professional life-style of decorum and subservient behavior. Rushing, in a study of "deference behavior" among psychiatric nurses, described how one individual will behave in a deferential manner toward another because of a relationship based on status difference.[6]

Nurses have long behaved in a deferential manner toward doctors, but this seems to be changing. No longer do all nurses pause to allow the doctor to precede them into a room. Only recently have nurses stopped rising and offering the doctor the chair they have conveniently warmed.

The psychiatrists, naturally, discussed the nurse-doctor relationship in some detail. This relationship was praised, questioned, skirted, avoided, and perhaps denied by them. Although the behavior patterns described by the psychiatrists were not specifically referred to as a relationship, the comments made were fairly concrete. Stein has described this relationship as a deadly serious game. He felt that the participants in this game were similar to high-wire acrobats, and that a slip resulted in severe penalties![7]

---

[6] Rushing, W. A.:Social influence and social-psychological function of deference: a study of psychiatric nursing. In Skipper, J. K., and Leonard, R. C., editors: Social interaction and patient care, Philadelphia, 1965, J. B. Lippincott Co., pp. 366–375.

[7] Stein, L. I.: The doctor-nurse game, Archives of General Psychiatry **16**:699, June 1967.

The nurse was seen by the psychiatrists quite frequently as supportive to the doctor. The nurse "helps the doctor as he examines patients, and she carries on some of the preliminary conversation with the patient as, 'How are you getting along?' and this kind of thing, and helps the doctor, which is traditional and is perfectly good." This helpfulness to the doctor was reinterpreted by another interviewed psychiatrist as meaning that the nurse sees the whole patient, as does the physician, and is more in tune with the physical as well as mental health aspects of the patient's care. The nurse was also viewed as being ego building to the doctor, because she accepts the physician in his role and respects his position. Another interviewee said he liked to take a nurse on a home visit with him because she was attuned to what the doctor needed. Another physician-director emphasized that a nurse is a good "second" person to accompany a physician to make a home visit. "Having a woman accompany a man makes sense."

The idea that by being helpful the nurse can increase the psychiatrist's self-esteem was described in vivid terms by one of the psychiatrists. He felt that the nurse who is flexible can learn this function quite easily. This psychiatrist introduced the problem of the skilled psychiatric nurse encountering the psychiatric resident. He felt that the nurse should interpret her role as, "Your job here is to teach this guy how to be as good as you are and not be too obvious about it." This same psychiatrist said that the article, "The Doctor-Nurse Game"[8] was required reading for nurses on his unit and jokingly remarked, "Sometimes we let the doctors read it, but not too often."

Gamesmanship in the psychiatric setting

The comments made by the latter interviewee were discussed many times by the Task Force. Questions often centered around the rules of the game used by doctors and nurses to communicate. Of special interest was the game itself and how it was played in the psychiatric setting. The rules seemed pretty basic but techniques observed in these settings varied. Most prevalent was the technique of offering analysis of each other's behavior instead of dealing with the problem. A favorite game of the psychiatrist was to respond to a remark made by the nurse with, "How do you feel about that?" This game is characterized by Loeb, who described staff interaction in the mental hospital as a struggle for status, power, and role identification. A technique used to deny status and role is to play the diagnostic or interpretive game. "When an individual tries to assert his status prerogatives and role responsibilities, it is relatively simple in this culture affectively to diminish the impact by projecting onto or into such a person feelings of hostility."[9]

---

[8] *Ibid.*
[9] Loeb, *op cit*, p. 308.

Further discussion and exploration by Task Force members revealed that nurses seem universally to accept the need to play the game. It was also understood that one had to learn the game quickly as a survival technique. Failure to play the game was seen by nurses to result in immediate loss in communication, inability to establish a working relationship with the doctor, ostracism, and frequently elimination.

The nurse-doctor relationship in psychiatry often assigns to the nurse the role of the mother figure. Psychiatry, which is based on a philosophy of symbols and associations, is quite free to assign the nurse the task of being the symbol of the ever-nurturing mother. The psychiatrists in the group saw the nurse as relating well in the home situation; in fact, better than the rest of the team members—perhaps because it is universally accepted that the woman's place is in the home. One of the Task Force members related an anecdote in which she was identified on her team, which was involved in family crisis treatment, as the member most qualified to assist a patient with housework.

This mothering role was also seen as a negative behavior of a nurse. The nurse was seen as being harmful to some patients if she provided too much nurturance. However, the mother role is not seen as harmful by all. For instance, this writer has experienced an unusual confrontation by a psychiatric resident who objected to the employing of a male nurse as head nurse on a ward. The resident based his opposition on the fact that *he* represented the father figure on the ward, and felt that he needed a female head nurse to serve as the mother figure for the nursing staff and patients. An interesting hypothesis, which has not been tested for validity, is that the male nurse is seen as threatening to the male psychiatrist in the eternal struggle for power on the psychiatric unit. The male nurse also destroys the rules of the doctor-nurse game, which is based partially on sexual roles.

Overdependency on the doctor was defined by the psychiatrists as a negative nurse-doctor relationship. Several of the interviewees were critical of the nurse who sat back and waited for direction from the physician. "If she sits back and waits for orders, as the classical order of a doctor-nurse relationship is, she is going to feel frustrated."

Another area described as dangerous in the nurse-doctor relationship was the nurse who modeled her function on the doctor's role. Most of the psychiatrists felt that nursing had contributions of its own to make rather than trying to be "little Freuds." The fact that nurses often aspire to be one-to-one therapists was seen as trying to mimic the psychiatrist's role.

It was suggested that the movement toward developing the community mental health center was a positive one for both doctors and nurses. This move could provide the opportunity to throw off the traditional, hospital-oriented roles of nurse and doctor. The community was seen as the new arena with no established ground rules (though this may be wishful thinking) where perhaps the game, which is useless and hindering, could die a natural death. It is hoped by all the authors of this book that the doctor, nurse, and other team members can develop healthy, mature, and productive relationships and will no longer need to play games.

A nurse is a nurse is a nurse—or the nurse we know and don't love

In their struggle to define the role of the nurse in the comprehensive community mental health center, the psychiatrists dealt first with the familiar. The conversation was filled with such words as "traditional" and "stereotype." These concepts were utilized both in a positive and a negative manner, often relating to the same behavior.

It was quite appropriate that the psychiatrists seemed at ease in discussing the nurse as she is found in the social setting of the inpatient service, since it is firmly established and the rules of the game are well known and accepted by all. Doctors and nurses are trained in the hospital, and it is in that arena that they establish their first relationships. The rightful, or "good," place for the nurse is in the hospital setting. The psychiatrists also were at ease in discussing the role of the public health nurse in the home of the patient. They were able to discern her functions as appropriate and acceptable, much the same as the hospital nurse. However, the hospital nurse and the public health nurse were both seen in roles that were nurturing to the patient and helpful to the doctor. (Or should it be helpful to the patient and nurturing to the doctor?) The authors submit that the psychiatrists were quite comfortable in discussing the nurse in her known role or, perhaps more aptly, in her "place." Once the discussion moved to placing the nurse on the center staff with functions similar to that of the rest of the team, things became more vague and diffuse.

How did the psychiatrists describe the attributes of the traditional nurse? The familiar themes of direct patient care, medication, and supervision of nonprofessionals were dominant. They felt the nurse had more time to spend with the patient and was better able to make observations, which she reported to the rest of the team. Almost all the psychiatrists emphasized that the nurse knew more and had more experience than any other team member (except the doctor) in dealing with a medicated patient. The nurse was also described as helpful in supervising the nonprofessional. Passivity, sitting back, being afraid to talk were all listed as negative traditional attributes by the psychiatrists. One said, "characteristically, she has been so ingrained with this somewhat passive position in relationship to other disciplines, [she] does have to work a little harder at overcoming her tendency to sit back." Another psychiatrist said that passive nurses have difficulty in relating to psychiatric residents because "they never get comfortable and are always looking to the doctor to give them the kind of support that they need, and he is not able to give it to them." This passivity of nurses was of interest to Loeb, who, in a study of social interaction in a mental hospital, analyzed tape recordings of conferences and meetings. He found that although psychiatrists complained that nurses did not speak up in meetings, in actuality they talked as much as the psychiatrists did but the psychiatrists had just not heard them.[10]

The tendency of the traditional nurse to mother the patients was brought out by the group as both good and bad. They felt that mothering was good for the newly admitted patient, but that it could be harmful to the patient on his way back to the community.

The nurse today recognizes the dilemma of conflicting expectations of others. She is expected to be aggressive but not too much so, since the doctor is still deserving of respect. She is expected to be nurturing but not too mothering. She is asked to be responsible for the supervision of one group, yet must switch roles and defer to the rest of the hierarchy. The nurse of today must shed the uniform of tradition and be ready to expose herself to criticism and rejection by persons who are more comfortable dealing with her in her inherited hospital setting, wearing her graying white uniform.

The nurse in the comprehensive community mental health center—or the nurse we don't know and are afraid to love

"Actually, we have never had reason to talk about the role of nursing in a mental health center" was how one psychiatrist began his remarks. His point was reflected in the discussion by several other group members. They found it difficult to focus on their expectations of the function of a nurse in a center, because prior to this interview they had no experience with the nurse other than in her hospital-oriented role. The nurse was seen as the most competent and most knowledgeable person in the center to observe, evaluate, report on, and supervise patients on medication. Several of the psychiatrists described how a nurse was helpful in a clinic or community setting in this capacity.

Another area discussed frequently was the home visit or home supervision of the patient. This nursing function was often referred to as the traditional role of the public health or visiting nurse. Most of the group members had had some involvement with a public health nurse and were able to see this model as useful for the nurse in the comprehensive community mental health center. They felt that the nurse was the most valuable person to go to the patient's home, even if it was only to remind the patient to come to the clinic. The nurse was also viewed as the most valuable team member to accompany the doctor when he made the home visit. There was no discussion about the possibility of the nurse being an active therapist in the patient's home or an activator of primary prevention.

---

[10] Loeb, *op cit*, p. 309.

The nurse was seen as a valuable member in the inpatient and partial-care settings of the community mental health center. The identification of the nurse with the patient who is in a hospital-like setting is so strong that she is usually seen as necessary to the function of that setting.

The fact that a nurse can often communicate most effectively with other nurses was regarded as an asset. The nurse in the center was seen as helpful in dealing with other nurses in the community, especially in hospitals, public health agencies, offices, and schools. It was suggested that the nurse might serve as a consultant to the other nurses.

One of the female psychiatrists displayed great insight in urging that the nurse not take the leftovers from other team members in the community clinic setting. She said that the nurse, because of her tendency to sit back and take orders, frequently did those tasks and often accepted those patients that other team members did not want. "I don't see the nurse simply taking what is left over after all of the professionals have their cut out of the patient's treatment."

Most of the members of this group, with perhaps one or two exceptions, were interested in "getting the nurses out of the hospital into the home." Those members who had experience with utilizing nurses in community programs were quite enthusiastic and supportive. One psychiatrist cautioned, however, that the program was still highly experimental. Their reservations were based on reality. They were concerned about the acceptance of the nurse into the hierarchy. In fact, one psychiatrist warned that if a nurse took the initiative instead of waiting to be told what to do she would "get burned" a few times.

The nurse was also seen as someone who often took on more than she could handle because of her willingness to please. They said that the nurse often received "unfair treatment" from other team members because she was requested to do things she felt "uncomfortable" about. Just as the licensed psychiatric technicians later warned us, the psychiatrists emphasized that the nurse who chose to serve on a mental health center team would have to undergo some unpleasant times. However, the point was made by one psychiatrist that the doctor who is relatively inexperienced in community mental health will also experience a period of being asked to do things he has never done before.

The nurse as a woman—or out in center field

In a recent Peanuts cartoon strip, Lucy, a feminist if there ever was one, says, "This is a male-dominated game . . . why should I take orders from that stupid manager? I'm just as good as he is! Why should I stand out here in center field? This is degrading, and I resent it!"[11] And if anyone is in center

---

[11] *Peanuts* by Charles M. Schulz. Copyright 1970 United Feature Syndicate.

field in the mental health game, it is the nurse. The interviewees all had comments about the nurse as a team member that reflected this. One psychiatrist believed that the nurse was the hardest working member of the team; in fact, she worked about a third harder than anyone else. Another psychiatrist referred to the discrepancy in salary between the nurse and other members of the mental health professions. The fact that the nurse is frequently assigned work and patients no one else wants was regarded as a problem for nurses in the mental health center by the psychiatrist group. Are the nurses usually assigned to these jobs because of their passive, mothering, feminine role? Yes, is the unanimous reply of the Task Force.

In an earlier part of this chapter it was mentioned that the group interviewed reinforced the idea that the nurse as a woman is complementary to the doctor as a man. The nurse was both praised and criticized for being passive, dependent, and waiting to be told what to do. The male-female or dominant-passive relationship prevalent in doctor-nurse relationships is obviously a question not often scrutinized in the work setting. It is avoided by both doctors and nurses.

It is our hypothesis that nurses are tired of assuming the feminine passive role assigned to them by the male (and sometimes female) physician. They are tired of being supportive to the ever-so-delicate male ego and are fed up with being the mother figure for everyone, including the doctor.

In a recent lecture entitled, "Women as a Minority Group," Elise Boulding, a sociologist, said, "There are women who are livid with rage in the same sense blacks are at being denied power to shape their lives in comparison with other groups—notably, men—in society." She went on further to describe this fury that women feel, "There is definitely a [desiring] of bloodletting, similar to colonized groups throwing off their masters."[12]

It is the thesis of this Task Force that the continuation of the nurse-doctor game will reinforce poor working relationships. The continuation of the iatrogenic problem of the suppressed fury of nurses who are regarded as inferior by the medical profession will result in inevitable rebellion. It is recognized that a new freedom can be established by throwing off the chains of tradition or by discarding the white uniform. When the need for games is over, both nurses and doctors (and all other mental health workers) can become mature, creative, and self-respecting. Nurses are demanding the same things all minority people are asking: establishment of their rights in society, the right to equal treatment, and freedom from prejudice.

How does a nurse get that way and solutions for it

The psychiatrists spent some time discussing the socialization of the nurse and had some opinions as to what made the nurse behave the way she did.

---

[12] Von Ende, Z.: Panel of women lashes alleged injustices in 'men's world', The Denver Post, Friday, May 1, 1970, Denver, Colorado.

Not unlike the old argument of heredity versus environment, the question has been asked as to what made nurses into the traditionally passive women they are.

Those interviewed pointed both to the system and to nursing education. There is some evidence that doctors and nurses share similar problems in dealing with the system and their education. One psychiatrist felt that education of the nurse was too broad and encompassing. There was a tendency, this psychiatrist said, to try to make the nurse an expert in all fields without enough basic skills for any. An example of this is the problem that occurs when a new registered nurse is assigned to supervise experienced psychiatric technicians. In this case the nurse was seen by the psychiatrist as woefully unprepared. This is not unlike the new intern who, as soon as he has M.D. after his name, is expected to be an experienced physician.

Others believed that there was too much emphasis placed on teaching nurses psychotherapeutic techniques. One psychiatrist urged nurses to "forget about Hildegard Peplau and the rest of them—you know, they're trying to be junior psychiatrists instead of what they can be best and that is effective nursing people." Still a third psychiatrist emphasized strongly that he saw no reason for nurses to be trained for one-to-one techniques; in fact, he was opposed to this idea.

The psychiatrists felt that level of preparation was important in determining what a nurse did in a community mental health center. It was believed that each nurse had the responsibility to apply whatever she had in the way of formal training. The nurse with a master's degree was seen as especially helpful in the areas of consultation, research, and education. One group member, however, cautioned that these areas were not "secrets" that were available only to the master's level nurse.

Too much emphasis was placed on levels of training and qualifications in all the mental health fields said one psychiatrist, who felt that mental health planners should concentrate on meeting manpower problems rather than being so concerned with staffing. This psychiatrist felt that if too much emphasis were placed on a person's educational preparation, "the patients might be left high and dry and still without what they might need." She spoke out quite freely and with a message to which nurses and other professionals should listen: "I think the nurse should work with whatever skills and training she has, be able to utilize consultation from others, be able to offer consultation to others, and in this way be realistic about the problems which are enormous, and we have to bring all kinds of imaginative thinking to bear on." She was quite explicit in her detailed explanation of what the nurse might do. She felt that the nurse needed "additional preparation in the form of experience in working with real problems, coping with real situations." This psychiatrist made explicit statements about what supervision is and what it is for. She said that the nurse needs "the proper kind of supervision early in the game. She needs supervision from her own discipline; she needs supervision from others; if she is to learn all she needs to learn, I think she should have some experience in supervising." She also said, "It may not be too wild, although it is a bit unusual, for a nurse to supervise a doctor in some kinds of situations where there is clear delineation of her skills and what he may need from her in the way of help."

The group felt that nurses, during the formative stages, were not only caught in the inflexible grip of nurse educators but also were trained in a setting that reinforced the rigid establishment of nursing—the hospital. This process, often referred to as "training," was seen as a mothering process of students by educators, of a holding back and/or down, and a lack of exposure to liberalizing influences.

Many studies have been done on the education of nurses. One interesting one was done by Krueger, who lived for a period of time with a group of student nurses. She found that the group she studied were considered good nurses by the faculty if they followed faculty expectations of behavior.[13] If one were to draw inferences from Krueger's study, it might be that nurses who were quiet and passive were rewarded by the faculty, and nurses who fought against the system were labeled by the faculty as "bad." Perhaps this is one causative agent in the end product, the passive nurse.

The system or hierarchy within the nursing profession itself was seen as a real hazard to the realization of the full potential of the nurse. As one participant said, "I think it is because there is so confounded much binding up of energies in various kinds of feuds and of jurisdictional disputes and all kinds of prima donna-like behavior that I think is most unbecoming that it reminds me very much of the rather encrusted state in which the American Psychiatric Association was at about the end of World War II."

The group felt that there was unnecessary bickering not only within the profession of nursing but also with other groups, such as the Licensed Psychiatric Technician. An analogy was drawn to the sparring relationship between psychiatrists and psychologists. This battle for power and status was seen as useless—a struggle in which the so-called helping professions battled with each other and neglected the patient.

If you care to accept it

A contemporary program on television starts the story with, "Your mission, if you care to accept it . . ." At times, the idea of nurses working effectively in the community mental health center is akin to an impossible mission.

What nursing has not faced is that while the community mental health center touts itself as new, unorganized, and flexible, in reality it is a social setting with carefully established ground rules. In their desire to be regarded

---

[13] Krueger, C.: Do bad girls become good nurses, Transaction, July/August 1968, pp. 31-36.

as untraditional, practitioners in community mental health centers are rejecting all that is traditional, and to many mental healthers the nurse continues to be identified with the hospital. Therefore, she is seen as the stereotype of one who cares for the sick. The nurse is viewed as the person who cares for the chronic, unwanted patient who has done something so terrible he must be segregated in a hospital.

The social system of the community mental health center could be considered a rigid one, and many mental health practitioners in this system display behavior similar to that of missionaries bringing salvation to a primitive society. Too often the program is based on what, in the judgment of the professional staff, is good for the consumer. If a nurse is accepted into this social system, she is frequently labeled the "doctor's helper" and is relegated to doing what the rest of the staff want to avoid.

Nursing, if it wishes to assume this impossible mission, must clearly recognize that by moving into the social system of the center, a change in the system is being made. If a nurse accepts lower status in an established hierarchy that externally considers itself democratic, equality of status is a mirage.

A question that one may pose is, are community mental health centers really willing to represent themselves as caring for those patients formerly sent to insane asylums? There is strong evidence[14] that the words *in*patient and *out*patient are symbolic of sickness and health—inpatient is associated with illness, weakness, and irresponsibility and outpatient is associated with wellness, healthiness, and responsibility.

If one lets one's fancies roam it could be supposed that part of the rejection of the nurse by the mental health center is related to the center's rejection of anything connected with the chronically ill. The nurse is questioning her exclusive role in caring for the weak and the sick, and is developing more concern for the person in the community. Should we explore this concept? Does the psychiatrist not want the nurse in the center because her presence somehow legitimizes the center's function of caring for the mentally ill, the sick, the chronic, the incurables?

Summary

This chapter in retrospect deals very little with the patient or with who gives care and how. It seems to center more around doctor-nurse relationships and the conflict that occurs when a fairly stable social hierarchy is disturbed. What is *status* in the hierarchy of mental health professionals? It is an interesting question. Is it the person who has the most intimate contact with the patient? No, because then the licensed psychiatric technicians would be at the top. Is it the type of thing a helper does, is that why the one-to-one

---

[14] Loeb, *op cit*, p. 307.

therapeutic relationship is zealously guarded by some psychiatrists as an animal would guard territorial rights? Certainly competence is one criterion mentioned as a measure of worth in the mental health hierarchy. However, being competent in one's profession doesn't pay off in money, status, or power.

What is it about the doctor-nurse relationship that propels doctors and nurses alike into continuous conflict? Nurses accuse doctors of being rigid, oppressive, and controlling. Doctors complain that nurses are rigid, passive, smothering, and controllable. One author discussed the problem with a psychiatrist friend who is active in community mental health. His reply was instantaneous. "What you have here is a neurotic marriage where one partner complains of being mistreated, beaten, abused, and the other partner complains that he beats because his partner demands it. Neither partner can bear to separate this neurotic pattern." Is that it? Is it necessary or possible to save this marriage? These are all questions which we, the Task Force, can't answer. We have left it to our readers to explore.

Chapter Four

LICENSED PSYCHIATRIC TECHNICIANS— A KICK FROM BEHIND

One of the last interviews that we conducted was with six licensed psychiatric technicians. They were employed, with one exception, at both of the State Hospitals in Colorado and all were graduates of the training programs for psychiatric technicians at those hospitals. The exception was a licensed psychiatric technician who at that time was enrolled in a mental health worker program at a local community college. The group was made up of both men and women and the participants had varying levels of responsibility.

In 1964, the first attempt was made to have a law passed for licensure of psychiatric technicians in Colorado.[1] When the law was not passed the first time, a campaign was begun by a dedicated and hardworking group of psychiatric technicians and their supporters. Regardless of some opposition from various power groups, such as the local psychologist and psychiatrist associations as well as some prominent nurse leaders, the law was passed in 1968. The prime supporter was the Colorado Nurses' Association. Mandatory licensure for all psychiatric technicians began in Colorado in 1969. The Colorado Psychiatric Technicians' Association has assumed responsibility for being the watchdog for its licensure law. Psychiatric technicians are licensed by the Colorado State Board of Nursing. For purposes of clarity, the licensed psychiatric technician is included as a mental health professional. Several of the members of the group we interviewed were officers of the National Association of Psychiatric Technology headquartered in California. This organization is the licensed psychiatric technicians' official organization of which the Colorado Psychiatric Technician Association is a constituent.

Length of experience is often one criterion for claiming expertise in one's field of endeavor. Status is often afforded to various subclasses according to tenure in the field. Of all the disciplines interviewed, the licensed psychiatric technicians probably had the most clinical experience collectively. The group's years of experience, if put on a continuum, would be over a century. The opinions of the licensed psychiatric technicians could be regarded as expert if one gave credit to their tenure in the field of caring for the mentally ill rather than their paper credentials. Historically, there has always been a caretaker in the institutions designed to care for the mentally ill, and nurses were, and still are, few in ratio to the caretaker group. Social workers and

---

[1] Hedges, F.: A brief history of the Colorado Psychiatric Technicians' Association. In Fuzessery, Z., editor, New frontiers in psychiatric technology, Second Annual Education Workshop of the Colorado Psychiatric Technicians' Association, Pueblo, Colorado, April 1969.

psychologists are even more recent additions to the scene. Patterson has commented on the evolution of the licensed psychiatric technician from this caretaker role: "Historically, I am told, the psychiatric technician was relegated to functioning in menial jobs which no person on the hospital staff could do or cared to do. I am sure ten years ago it seemed impossible that the old image of the untrained and uncaring attendant would ever be shaken. Currently, however, it would be foolhardy, if not impossible, to try to have a relevant treatment program without a force of trained psychiatric technicians."[2] It is no wonder that the licensed psychiatric technician of today does not always stand in awe of all the latecomers to the field of giving direct care to the mentally ill.

These licensed psychiatric technicians were not afraid to say what they thought; they had a sense of pride and worth. As one member said, "We're psychiatric technicians. We think we're damn good ones and damn proud of it." Perhaps if one were to seek out the word most descriptive of the attitude of the psychiatric technician it would be *down to earth*. Absent were phrases such as "coordinator," "caring," and "helping." More often heard were "supervision," "management," and "teaching." Most of the group addressed themselves to the inpatient service, although they also had ideas to contribute about community mental health care. The licensed psychiatric technician, for the most part, has not become a part of the comprehensive community mental health center, but is familiar to the inpatient service. In describing the functional role of the nurse in the inpatient service, the licensed psychiatric technicians emphasized that giving of medications was perhaps the most unique nursing function, but that the following functions were also an integral part of the nurse's role: (1) meeting the emotional needs of patients, (2) managing the environment for both staff and patients, (3) identification of nursing goals in relation to specific nursing care problems and formulating care plans, (4) relating to and communicating with other team members, (5) co-therapist in group therapy, (6) directing of psychodrama, (7) teaching technicians, and (8) anticipating and predicting means by which patients could learn how to cope with crisis after hospitalization.

Of all the professional groups interviewed to that time, the psychiatric technician group saw the role of the nurse to be much the same as their own. In fact, they saw very little difference in function and responsibility. One said, "I think I see the nurse participating in a lot of the same types of things that I do as a psychiatric technician." Another said, "Except for medications, they do pretty much the same things we do." One technician felt that a nurse was socialized to her role: "After she is on duty for a while she gets to be practically like the rest of us. I mean that you would have a hard time telling

---

[2] Patterson, L.: Whose values?, Colorado Psychiatric Technicians' Association, Feb. 1970.

who is who." They did not have to guess and hint at what nurses did and should do; they knew from long and intimate experience in working with nurses caring for patients. What about this similarity? Both licensed psychiatric technician and the nurse were hospital oriented. Both tended to view patients as sick and were able to conceptualize mental disorders as having a disease base that was susceptible to diagnosis, treatment, and perhaps cure. Is this the reason that it is difficult to tell who is who? The sharing of similar training and similar functions has seemed to lead the licensed psychiatric technicians to visualize the sharing of similar problems. The questions of who actually gives direct patient care and who spends the most time with the patient were perceived by the licensed psychiatric technicians as being themselves rather than the nurse. They saw the nurse spending more of her time relating to other team members about patient care rather than giving direct patient care.

Who gets the August vacations?

The licensed psychiatric technicians gave several clues as to who is who. The nurse is the one who ends up "worrying about who is getting Sunday off and August vacations." By some of their statements, it could be inferred that the licensed psychiatric technician felt that nurses were getting caught up in an administrative bind. It was pointed out that while nurses expounded the belief that real nursing was direct patient care, they tended to seek out—or were at times pushed into—management duties. In the opinion of the group the nurse is the person on the team who makes out schedules, plans assignments, supervises the nonprofessional, and gives medications. This group saw the licensed psychiatric technician as the person most available for direct patient care and perhaps the best person to provide this care. They felt the nurse should admit she is not available for this function. Amusingly enough, the nurse was perceived by some technicians to be frustrated. "Perhaps the fact that they have to keep track of medications and usually there are not as many nurses and they have to rotate more frequently, a lot of times their role isn't as expanded as the technicians, and I think it can be quite threatening to the nurses." One person said, "This is not right. It is a misuse of ability, misplacing that person from what she has been trained for." This theme of being responsible for the "dynamic duo" of inpatients and medications seemed to have been a unilateral interpretation by all the professions interviewed. In Chapter 7 mention is made by one psychiatrist that a nurse's strength actually lies in these areas of management, knowledge of medicines, coping techniques, and supervision of nonprofessionals. In discussions about these realities, we felt that nurses as a group need to reevaluate their strengths and perhaps develop them as attributes rather than burdens. However, we also found ourselves wondering why the managerial model has become to so many persons our modus operandi. (In Chapter 8 this point is discussed from a different frame of reference.) This may be the price we pay for an amorphous role!

The new grad phenomenon

When the licensed psychiatric technician began to describe and criticize the phenomenon of the new graduate nurse being assigned to supervise the more experienced licensed psychiatric technician, both the interviewees and interviewers were on familiar ground. A quality of nostalgia crept into the discussion as the familiar problems created by this too common situation were again reviewed. The old frustrations were reexamined. One licensed psychiatric technician described the experience as a painful one for both the nurse and technician. Another believed that nurses should have more training in supervision to prepare them to assume leadership and management roles. He felt the difficulties in supervisory relationships of licensed psychiatric technicians and nurses were related to poor training of nurses for leadership roles. Others, such as Ethel Bonn, have also recognized the dilemma in which the new nurse finds herself when she moves into the mental health setting. Dr. Bonn finds this to be a problem not only for nursing and licensed psychiatric technicians but also for the mental health center. She describes this problem as the difficulty the new registered nurse experiences when she must supervise licensed psychiatric technicians who know more about the center and its function than she does. Dr. Bonn perceives this to be more a problem of lack of knowledge of the center as a society or system than as a lack of theoretical knowledge in the clinical area.[3]

A theory proposed by one of the authors of this book, that the new nurse who enters the psychiatric or other setting and experiences the pressure of the system is often a victim of the Peter Principle—"In a hierarchy every employee tends to rise to his level of incompetence."[4] The new nurse who is placed in a leadership position by the hierarchy may be perceived as incompetent by virtue of inexperience both by herself and by those she supervises. Her incompetence in the managerial role is as much the responsibility of the hierarchy as it is the nurse.

The nurse with a master's degree seemed to be valued by the licensed psychiatric technician. They were emphatic in seeing the nurse with a master's degree as more helpful in comparison to other nurses to the nonprofessional. They wanted the benefit of her knowledge, guidance, and experience. They definitely do not want her to "waste" her skills "doing." Perhaps some of the technicians' feelings stemmed from the fact that during their training most

---

[3] Bonn, E. M.: A therapeutic community in an open state hospital. Administrative—therapeutic links, Hospital and Community Psychiatry **20**:270, Sept. 1969.

[4] Peter, L. J., and Hull, R.: The Peter principle—why things always go wrong, New York, 1969, William Morrow & Co., Inc., p. 25.

of the instructors were nurses who had master's degrees. It is our impression that the feelings of the licensed psychiatric technicians about nurses are ambivalent. On one hand they say the nurse is the same as the licensed psychiatric technician in function and role (except for the giving of medications), yet they berate the nurse for her lack of leadership and management skills. A recurring theme was that the nurse, in failing to assume more aggressive leadership, was stifling the licensed psychiatric technician. Is it possible that the licensed psychiatric technician, by asking the nurse to provide more leadership, is indirectly asking for a more encompassing role in direct patient care for themselves?

Who are we?

Those interviewed raised the familiar and poignant cry of "We have lost our identity." As they continued to discuss who does what, they felt that the interchange of roles and function served to create some confusion and a sense of loss in knowing what one's specialty was. With the coming of the mental health worker to community mental health, there were again questions of how did everyone fit into the pattern. Who did what? S. B. Schiff has said that to deal with the frustrations and problems that occur with role blurring, the team needs to develop role sharpening. He felt that it was important to ". . . not perceive all staff with members equal in performance and function."[5] Perhaps the licensed psychiatric technicians were asking nurses to redefine their role, especially in areas of leadership management, teaching, supervision, and administration of medicine. There seemed to be some indication that if nursing could delineate function, the licensed psychiatric technicians themselves could see more clearly their place in the system. It seemed to us that mental health nurses were asked by licensed psychiatric technicians to relinquish their totem of direct patient care and recognize that the licensed psychiatric technicians were more involved with the patient. If nurses did this, then the licensed psychiatric technician could define *direct patient care* as their role.

Where the community is

The group had a strong concept of community. All of them had been involved in some facet of direct community services, such as aftercare, foster home placement, and agency consultation. They were able to discuss community services based upon actual experiences. They brought up and discussed salient points not even considered by other professional groups. For example, they aired their views about community psychiatry and community relationships. They have not swallowed so quickly the platitude of "keep the patient

---

[5] Schiff, S. B.: A therapeutic community in an open state hospital. Administrative framework for social psychology, Hospital and Community Psychiatry **20**(9):22, Sept. 1969.

in the community." As one technician put it, "We may be trying to operate community psychiatry with programs that have been in existence and accepted for fifty to seventy-five years." They have recognized that "The community pronounces the patient guilty before we ever see him." They go on further and describe that one must realize that your patient can tell you, "I could care less about that community. As far as I am concerned they can go to hell in that community." To community psychiatry enthusiasts, the technician warns "psychiatry today calls [certain behaviors] a hundred different things and classifies them diagnostically when to the community, the patient is a behavior problem." Regardless of the language and the classification that professionals use, the patient is seen as exhibiting behavior that is unacceptable in that community. The technicians identified this area as "going to be one great challenge of the nurse going into those communities and working with these particular problems." One technician said, "This is going to be new to most individuals [nurses] that have been used to working in operating rooms, pediatric wards, or something." The "something," one could speculate, means traditional institutional psychiatric settings as well as general hospital settings.

The technicians had concrete and realistic suggestions for community mental health centers. They felt the aim of the center should be to put "the money where the patient is—not the patient where the money is." They discussed the sometimes difficult task of returning the patient to a community that felt it had solved problems by sending the patient to the hospital. This need for closer relationships between law and police authorities and the need for better understanding of socially unacceptable and deviant behavior was seen as being vital in a truly comprehensive community mental health center. They felt that because many of the patients seen in the institutional settings were community rejects because of unacceptable behavior, there should be greater emphasis on programs for teaching the social deviant better behavior.

Get your feet wet

The licensed psychiatric technicians saw themselves sharing with the nurse extremely difficult progress along the path from the hospital to the community. They felt that they still had the same obstacles and barriers to overcome that the nursing profession has already experienced. The nurse and the technician are lowest in status on the mental health team. They are generally ambivalent about the caretaker role that is thrust upon them by other professionals. Technicians share with nurses the assignment to the chronic patient, the geriatric patient, and the character disorder—the group of patients often referred to among mental healthers as the "dumping syndrome." The one difference that is outstanding is that the technicians see nurses as one of the barriers to their being accepted in the community mental health center. The nurse is in the way of the psychiatric technician in his movement into community mental health. One technician put it succinctly, "we can't go ahead unless nurses go ahead," and then urged nurses to go ahead. The licensed psychiatric technicians offered suggestions and advice to nurses about working in community mental health centers. "They need to get their feet wet. They're not even accepted yet." The licensed psychiatric technician warned us that "nurses have an awful lot of work to do to even get their foot in the door." They urged nursing to "take a leading step forward even though you might get slapped in the face for it." "Slaps" are usually related to demanding equal status in the hierarchy, such as equal pay for equal education or moving into the therapist role. In spite of these warnings of grim possibilities, the licensed psychiatric technician is eager for the nurse to establish a foothold in the community mental health center. The reason for urging this push is clear. The licensed psychiatric technician sees nurses as their precursor. They realize that nursing has to be accepted and sanctioned before the licensed psychiatric technician can be recognized as a valid performer in the hierarchy of mental health professionals. They emphasized the value of preparation and not "just the simple fact that a nurse has a bachelor's degree qualifies her to go ahead and practice psychiatric nursing." The licensed psychiatric technician pointed out that additional preparation and experience might prevent the nurse from being "clobbered easily." No one in the Task Force questioned from whence the clobbering came, but in rereading the transcript, it seemed reasonably clear that the clobbering would come from either the community or from other members of the mental health team.

The go-between

Current mental health action programs urge and stipulate that indigenous workers be used in the existing programs. There has been encouragement for community involvement. The licensed psychiatric technician, aide, or nonprofessional could be considered to be a precursor to the currently popular indigenous worker. Like the currently involved worker, the licensed psychiatric technician is usually recruited from the community in which the hospital (or insane asylum) is located. They are paid as low a wage as possible and often more for brawn than brain. These nonprofessionals often become the go-between, the gate-keepers between the hospital and the community. Often they provide the "good will" for the hospital or perhaps the "bad name" by just being willing to work in such a place. These workers are the ones who are often accused of being nonprofessional, of becoming involved with patients and families. Nurses sometimes slip too, in becoming "too familiar" with patients, but it is almost an expectation that the aides would do this also. These techniques now thought of as innovative and previously unheard of for professionals have long been used by aides and technicians in giving patient care.

So what else is new?

There has been greater emphasis in psychiatry on physical closeness with patients. The sharing of a social activity with a patient by a physician, social worker, or psychologist is regarded as an innovative technique. The nurse and technician have been doing this for years. One of the authors recently observed an incident in which a patient was taken to her home on a visit by a psychiatric resident and nurse. At home this patient assumed the hostess role and served coffee and cookies. Twenty-four hours earlier she had had to be physically restrained in a seclusion room because she was biting herself. This incident points out what both nurses and technicians have told other members of the mental health team: behavior differs depending on the setting. In a hospital setting the patient is permitted (encouraged) to act crazy; in the patient's normal setting the crazy behavior often disappears.

It is amazing to us that some of the "innovations" have been in use for years in Europe. Home care is a good example. Here in the United States as soon as a psychiatrist steps into the home, the popular magazines tout it as an untried technique.

In agencies and institutions it was common for patients to be addressed by their first name, nurses and attendants by their last name, and doctors by their title. It is now common for everyone but the doctors and perhaps the social workers to be addressed by his first name.

It is hoped that the mental health team can utilize the nurse and technician in closing the social distance between the doctor and the patient so that a more therapeutic understanding can be established. The nurse and the technician are the only members of the mental health team who share with the patient his daily 24-hour routine. The nurse and technician are aware not only of how the patient sleeps, but also where he sleeps, what he eats and where, what the patient does or does not do most of the day.

A few examples will illustrate the distance between the physician and the patient. We have observed several occasions on which a physician or social worker called for a nurse or technician for assistance when the patient was nauseated or had to go to the bathroom. In addition, we have heard a patient tell a physician he was hungry and the doctor tell the patient to ask the nurse. Another similar personal experience occurred when a physician called one of the authors to forcibly remove a squalling infant from the arms of a schizophrenic and possibly homicidal mother who had come into the emergency clinic. Unfortunately, these examples fit all too well under the heading "So What Else Is New?" We will comment in more depth on this type of behavior in the last part of this book.

Implications for nursing

Unique in the total exchange of ideas between the licensed psychiatric technicians and the Task Force was the lack of defensiveness. There was an atmosphere of mutual understanding and acceptance, with perhaps a bit of misery loves company thrown in. There was little, if any, female-male sparring, and the question of sexual roles never arose despite the fact that this was a mixed group. The sameness of role and function and perhaps the lower status in relation to other disciplines gave the technicians and nurses a feeling of sharing. Shared problems were identifiable as (1) lack of acceptance by community mental health centers, (2) assignment of role of caretaker, (3) identification with caretaking of the chronic patient no one else wants to accept, and (4) inequitable salary scales. However, the technicians saw nurses as an obstacle to their own fight for recognition. They gave a loud and clear warning to the nursing profession. In referring to themselves and other mental healthers, they said, "You're going to have rebellion from these groups— you have to hear their side and feel their feelings." It is the authors' opinion that the perception of the psychiatric technician is generally true; that the nurse of today is too willing to please and accepts the dump without objection. Nurses, generally, have lacked the militant spirit that is necessary in dealing with the overt and covert rejection by community mental health centers.

Chapter Five

THE SOCIAL WORKERS LOOK

In this chapter the ideas expressed reflect the views of a group of six social workers regarding the role of the nurse, her basic preparation, and ways to implement the ideas they had discussed. The chapter also reflects the views of the participant-observers concerning the atmosphere and nonverbal communication and presents our interpretation of the tape recording transcript.

The group of social workers consisted of two men and four women. At the time of the interview they were all employed in community mental health centers or public psychiatric facilities and had been active in social work in various areas and at various levels for a number of years.

The interview situation seemed to create pressure for the participants. For example, they appeared anxious about the use of the tape recorder, and although they had received in advance a set of questions for discussion, they did not appear to know what was expected. Possibly some of the stress was related to a personal reaction in searching for their own identities, which had been stimulated by the questions to be considered. They experienced more difficulty than other groups in differentiating between a public health and a psychiatric nurse as is evidenced at times in the text which follows. For some reason, the public health model was seen as the "good" nurse, while the psychiatric nurse was seen as typifying the "bad" institutional model. The institutional model in all instances was viewed negatively. There was obviously no understanding of the fact that most nurses with baccalaureate degrees had some exposure to public health nursing, whereas the nurse who had received a diploma from a nursing school had little if any.

After an introductory period and a rather candid description of the rationale for the study, there was a long silence which was fractured by the voice of one of the male social workers. His opening statement was, "I could start off to break the tensions here." This was an adequate description and seemed to set the mood for the session. The theme that recurred throughout the interview was: "You can make a social worker out of a nurse, but you can't make a nurse out of a social worker." During the session several questions were asked regarding the preparation of the nurse for such activities as one-to-one and group therapy. Later in the discussion, when it had been established that specialists in psychiatric nursing were being prepared and had developed skills in these activities, the social workers then said that these particular skills were ones that anyone could learn. It was reminiscent of an Old Salem law: a stone was tied around the neck of a person accused of witchery and he was tossed into a well to decide the question of his guilt. If the individual drowned he was proclaimed innocent; if he bobbed up he was guilty and consequently burned at the stake. This bind of being damned if you do or damned if you don't is still very much with us.

Nursing education—for what

An important element in the discussion was the lack of information the social workers had regarding nursing education, function, and role.

In addition to a lack of basic knowledge relating to the difference between diploma education and baccalaureate education previously mentioned, the social work group evidenced almost total ignorance of preparation at the master's level for psychiatric nurses. Such questions as: "Do they have orientation in the transference and counter-transference elements of treatment and this sort of thing? It has been my impression that they haven't!" (This particular statement leads one to believe that this individual feels that if you don't dig Sigmund, you can't understand the action.) Another social worker underlined this impression by relating it to the large amount of case discussion in the present mental health center setting. It was inferred that the nurses felt awkward in a setting of verbal conceptualization and could not enter case discussion and planning unless they were at least at the master's level with more experience. Actually, that statement does have some validity, as is often evidenced in a multidiscipline case conference when many nurses have been observed to be passive participants.[1] However, she went on to say that it is difficult to assess the nurse's skills as to whether they are due to training, experience, personality, understanding of people, or something else entirely. Could this particular problem be one that is shared by all of the health professions?[2]

The blight on white

The social workers described the traditional, institutional nurse as inactive, nonparticipating, using control negatively, being task oriented, and lacking independent functioning. These observations seem to express a definite relationship between social workers' perception of the hospital role of the nurse and the absence of nurses in many mental health centers. One social worker said that his experiences and negative memories handicapped his looking at nurses in relation to the more flexible setting of the mental health center. He continued, "That's why I've been so anxious to get the nurse out of the uniform because then I could accept her in a new role. While she was in uniform, I thought of her as a restrictive passive-aggressive mother." Their conclusion

[1] Lamb, R. H., Heath, D., and Downing, J. J. In Bowen, P., Wygant, L. S., Heath, D., and others, editors: Handbook of community mental health practice, San Francisco, 1969, Jossey-Bass, Inc., Publishers, p. 181.
[2] *Ibid*, p. 73.

was, "Let's define a different role for the nurse—a more dynamic function than the traditional, since the nurse in her traditional role is not particularly valuable to us in the community setting."

Another social worker had brought up the question of nurses wearing a uniform in connection with a research project that was being conducted at a large public health agency. The result of the survey, he reported, was that the public health nurse wanted her uniform for many reasons, but the most common reasons were (1) as an entree into the home and (2) for protection. He discussed the responsibility of administration for providing an environment that was not too restrictive, so that the individual could grow in the position. He cited the administrative attitude regarding uniforms and said, "For example, some people have gone out of uniform, and patients and staff alike are concerned about this unmasking of certain impulses that may come out when the nurse is not in the traditional uniform." As a more aggressive group of "mothers," we would like to respond to these remarks. Out of uniform and into trouble—if you wear the uniform you are considered rigid; if you wear civilian clothes, you are viewed as lacking role identity or as a sex maniac. It provokes thought as to whether the wearing of a uniform creates a communication barrier.

People will be people

A problem that is now facing mental health facilities in relation to role extension or blurring is how best to use the unique attributes of the workers and get the most from each without duplication. The social workers felt that it should be based upon the worker's personality, using a certain social worker or a certain nurse according to his individual comfort index and specialized skill. This point was in turn related to the administrative structure of a community mental health center. What they saw as the administrative responsibility of the center was idealistic but not beyond the realm of possibility. They saw the center as having the responsibility for providing an administrative atmosphere in which the employee would have the freedom to try working in a variety of areas. The individual would then be free to pursue in depth the area in which his expectations are most adequately met. They felt that a center which had policies limiting the role of the nurse or any other worker was severely restrictive both to the individual and to performance. As Downing states, "granting of autonomy always poses a multitude of problems."[3] In order to grant rational autonomy, the capabilities of the worker ought to be known. Unfortunately, the social worker has little idea about what the nurse is equipped to do. A statement to this effect was made: "Are there role levels among nurses? For example, would you hire a psychiatric nurse

---

[3] Lamb, Heath, and Downing, L.: *op cit*, p. 26.

for inpatient service and a public health nurse for outpatient services and half and half for partial hospitalization?" A pertinent question may be: What would be helpful in acquainting the social worker with the nurse, her education, and her potential role? A growing number of nurses are receiving master's degrees. The social worker may not realize that the nurse might also have had specialized training which, in some ways, may be similar to his own. One of the social workers felt it would be fascinating to ask why people go into the various health fields. She felt it would be revealing to compare the present with ten years ago because of the changes that had taken place. She said that she didn't choose nursing because she "didn't want to get messed up with bedpans and all the rest of it. I wanted to relate without getting involved with that sort of thing. Nursing would never appeal to me at all." One of our authors had difficulty restraining herself from saying aloud that from the bedpan we had learned the anal phase of development. Another social worker added, "Is one reason people are attracted to the nursing profession because the role has been closely defined with an authoritative person always hovering over that you could blame everything on?"

It takes one to know one

It was apparent that the social workers in the group had had limited experience working with nurses. Some had more experience than others, but all based their ideas, feelings, and conclusions on their experiences with individual nurses. Whether they saw nurses as useful or not had more to do with the reaction of the social worker to an individual nurse. The social workers' own educational background plus the theory or theories of human behavior within which they worked were involved as well. The social workers repeatedly emphasized that they regarded understanding of transference and counter-transference important for any member of the mental health team. One social worker called the group's attention to the fact that they were speaking from a psychoanalytic frame of reference which, he said, was "his bag" but that in the comprehensive community mental health center "we are finding that many modalities of treatment are being used, and you might find that other staff members may very well choose or prefer another frame of reference as their treatment modality." He added that as a training experience for mental health professionals, the comprehensive community mental health center would be lacking if many therapy modalities were not present for the trainee to explore. The Task Force wonders if we should not also consider the patients' responses to the different modalities of therapy? Sometimes we wonder if only nurses think about what happens to the patient.

The social worker who had inferred that if a person were not "Freudenized," he or she might not understand the "action," stated that even though she felt the analytical frame of reference was important, she had seen value in the public health model of prevention. She further explained that this model was effective in working with wellness, particularly in the context of the family. "I think the public health nurse can seek out a patient in the larger context where sometimes a person trained in the analytic approach has trouble, and I think the mental health center demands this perception of the individual." This particular statement seemed to indicate the inadequacy of the psychoanalytic approach as the prime modality for treatment in a community mental health center, and this inadequacy does indeed seem evident in coping with the majority of problems presented by patients and families in community mental health centers.

In this corner with or without uniform and in this corner with or without Freud

A social worker who stated she had had one experience working with a nurse in the psychiatric field felt that the nurse was a definite asset to the mental health team. She believed the nurse was helpful at those times when the team doctor was not available for consultation and she was able to turn to the nurse for an understanding of medications, reactions, side effects, and physical problems.

In response to the question concerning the basic preparation needed by the nurse to function in the community mental health center, social workers seemed to agree that in addition to basic nursing education and master's education, about which they knew little, the nurse should have three specific attributes. (1) She should know her book well. She should know the psychiatric syndromes, have a frame of reference (preferably the analytical frame) that would enable her to make a sound diagnosis, to set up a treatment plan, and to follow through with the treatment plan, (2) she should know herself well, and (3) she should know her limitations in terms of therapeutic capacity. She should feel free to consult with and ask for help from other mental health professionals. In addition, they felt it would be valuable for the nurse to have experience working with psychiatric syndromes in a hospital setting. Such work would allow her to be more comfortable with these same types of emotional illnesses in the community and would enable her to assess and evaluate the patient's strength as well as his pathology.

One male social worker from a large state-operated agency felt that because he had found the public health nurse to be flexible and capable of independent functioning, it would be best to start with a public health nurse and "build" the other attributes into the person through interdisciplinary training. Another social worker also felt that public health training, plus a community orientation and working with other agencies and disciplines, was necessary as basic educational and professional preparation for the nurse in a comprehensive community mental health center. She believed that such knowledge should be a part of the education of all health professionals who work in centers. Another social worker was concerned with the nurse's need for skills and training in individual and group therapy. And yet another stated that one of the most valuable contributions of the psychiatric nurse is in the management of psychiatric patients who are in a general hospital setting. This nurse can assist the nonpsychiatric nurse in managing these patients. This need was expressed by a social worker employed by a large state general hospital that has a comprehensive psychiatric service and whose emergency service for such cases was part of the general emergency room services of the hospital. The nurse would be assigned consultative, educational, and supervisory functions. The same social worker felt that a unique contribution of the nurse was working with patients and their families on an outpatient basis.

The community—is it what the professional wants to treat?

One aspect of care mentioned only briefly by the group was the need of the professional community to work with people whose cultural backgrounds are different from their own. A problem that we hear discussed frequently is the difficulty encountered in understanding the behavior of patients who are from different cultural backgrounds. The charge is often made that professionals frequently impose their own middle-class cultural norms on the patient. For example, one incident mentioned concerned a psychiatrist who told the social worker that because he had a middle-class background, he was not sure that he could work with the patients the public health nurse was bringing in. The staff discussed the problem, and the psychiatrist reluctantly agreed that he needed help. The social workers pointed out that public health nurses do not have this handicap. The house may smell and may be a highly undesirable place to visit, but the nurse may, in fact, like the patient. The social worker who shared this information felt that the nurse could be helpful in assisting the psychiatrist to overcome his negative feelings and readjust his thinking so that he could deal effectively with people whose values are different from his own.

Little Blue Riding Hood

The social workers found public health nurses a tremendous and willing resource for dealing with chronic patients and patients with character disorders. They saw no role conflict in this area, as they made it clear they did not want this role. One of the male social workers reported that at his center, which has a staff of seventeen professionals, there were no psychiatric nurses. He said that the practical reason was that they had used and probably will continue to use public health nursing services. His mental health center had cooperated closely with public health nurses for some time and found that many of the public health nurses, with consultation and support, had been adequate for services within the community. He said further that this does require consultation and staff education for nurses, since not all public health nurses are sufficiently trained to handle all types of work. At that point, he belatedly expressed the hope that some day one or two psychiatric nurses would be added to the staff of that mental health center. Earlier in the session he had apologized for not including psychiatric nurses in the center's original grant request or on their team. The silent response of the Task Force to this was, "Oh, thanks a lot, big brother, for allowing psychiatric nurses in your mental health center. Are the public health nurses you have used on strike? Would you hire a mental health nurse to deal with chronic patients? What would happen if the mental health nurse saw her role differently; would she be allowed to see her role differently? It is sad that chronic patients are viewed as unwanted because these are patients who really need the care of everyone on the team, not just the person who happens to be on the bottom rung of the ladder in the health hierarchy at the time."

Nurses work with sickness—social workers, wellness

Part of the social workers' wish to delegate the care of the chronic patient to the nurse may be due to what they had observed regarding the types of patients with whom nurses seem to choose to work. They felt that nurses select sick patients, but when the patient moves toward a state of wellness the nurse is willing to give the care of the patient over to a member of another discipline. They said that nurses select patients with physical problems, psychosomatic illnesses, dependency needs, chronic illnesses, or patients who are members of the lower socioeconomic class and have many complicated problems. They saw the nurse as the team member who tended to stick with patients with the least optimistic prognosis; the patient who is least likely to get well; the patient who other team members would have dismissed long before as unresponsive. They also saw nurses as being more comfortable in a structured situation in which there is an authoritative person who could assume the responsibility as well as the blame.

Little Blue Riding Hood rides again

The subject of the chronic, poorly motivated patient's need for care was discussed at length with the social workers because it had so frequently been referred to as an integral part of the nurse's role. Their response to the question of why greater effort was not made on behalf of the chronic patient by the entire team was a self-enlightened answer: "When there are a lot of people needing help, it is simple and natural to take the seventy-five percent who really want to work with you, who know what we are there for, and so forth." This leaves a question about the other twenty-five percent. These seem to be the patients that are referred to the public health nurse. Perhaps we could better explore this question by asking the public health nurses who have been working with this twenty-five percent how to plan and how to set realistic goals. This statement was followed by a comment from the other male social worker. "I have to agree, that probably we have found, in general, the flexibility of the public health nurse to establish realistic goals has been far superior to the flexibility of the so-called psychiatric nurse. I think this may stem somewhat from the training base from which some of the psychiatric nurses come. I guess what I am saying is that the psychiatric nurse who is only institutionally trained is sort of task-oriented, whereas the public health nurse and an experienced psychiatric nurse is more process-oriented in that she sees herself in relation to the whole bit about problem-solving." The confusion seemed to center around what nurse, from what background—even to the point of what or to whom did the term "nurse" refer. Most of the members of the Task Force would regard this man's concept of the psychiatric nurse as narrow. He seemed to be idealizing the public health nurse as being a Little Blue Riding Hood—and assigning only her to the smelly house. The public health nurse's role in prevention was never mentioned.

The bedpan image and its effect on other disciplines

As a group we do not question the effect of the institutional model. Most of the social workers emphasized the nurse's functioning in a hospital environment and therefore saw her as being prepared to function primarily in the traditional way in a hospital setting. The problem of shifting the frame of reference from the hospital to the community one is not unique to the psychiatric nurses; the struggle exists among other members of the psychiatric community team as well. For example, in this discussion the social workers brought up the fact that administration of the community mental health center is generally taken to be a medical responsibility, the psychiatrists' jurisdiction. They brought out several problems they had seen as a result of the decision to allocate a medically and clinically trained person to a managerial position. They concluded that he was called upon to be many kinds of persons, to wear many hats. In certain tasks, because of his education, he performed adequately; in other tasks, because of a lack of experience and education, he was incompetent. They suggested that he could involve other members of the team in sharing their attitudes and points of view so that an effective, comprehensive community mental health program could be built. Nursing shares with other disciplines the urgent need to define its practice and role in dealing with emerging national health problems. The fact that the professionals themselves are resistive demonstrates the existence of some deeply set attitudes about the nature of professional roles. We have progressed, but clearly we have a long way to go.

What educational bag does the mental health team need?

After some discussion about a more functional, dynamic role for the nurse, the question arose: Is there a need for four separate educational programs for members of the mental health team if the graduates function in similar ways? Are there areas and professional skills basic to the four disciplines?

They considered the possibility of having a basic course for mental health workers, after which each person would select his particular area of study. This led to a discussion of an associate in arts degree for a mental health worker who will, in time, according to one social worker, replace nurses, social workers, and psychiatric technicians. These remarks seemed to generate some anxiety, and a second response to the question regarding preparation for nurses was made: "This brings up the question of who you are training and for what, and what difference is it going to make anyway." It is hard to keep from wondering if the threat of nurses coming into the community mental health center is so great to the social workers that they are willing to settle for a complete loss of identity for all specialized groups.

A model model

When discussing the model for delivery of mental health service, the group concluded that there is a need to question the present medical model and to see if other models (such as the educational or public health model) might not be superior. "Sometimes we feel inadequate, as our roles modify, because someone expects something of us that might not be realistic at this point." This statement was made by a social worker to emphasize the value of a professional education for the nurse starting in the mental health center. He felt that this was valuable because as the roles of members of the team began to expand, "you've got to be very secure within yourself in that particular role because it is going to be challenged, and unless you feel pretty good about being a nurse, you won't have room for expansion." Relating this to other disciplines he said, "We find professionals who can't stand this independence, can't stand the challenge, and do sort of wither away until they are dismissed." One interesting point added here was that the professional is first dismissed by the patient and finally by the co-workers. Could it be that the peer group feels insecure to some extent without the limits, standards, or knowledge of the job and is unable to evaluate its own performance? The sensitivity model was discussed and it was pointed out that sensitivity may develop an awareness, but when problems arise, sensitivity alone does not provide continuity and consistency; professional identity is needed as well. This led to a philosophical discussion of why people choose a particular field of endeavor. What influences their choice to become nurses rather than social workers? Are the characteristics believed to be typical of nurses or social workers present in the individual prior to his decision to become a nurse or a social worker, or are these characteristics the result of training and education? The social workers were very much aware that in the area of salary (equal pay for equal work) there was a rather large gap. However, the salary for a job with defined and specific responsibilities depends upon the discipline classification of the individual filling the position. This issue was not discussed further and no suggestions for change, resolutions, or recommendations were made.

How does one find complementary roles, especially where roles have not been explicitly differentiated from each other? (The doctor can rest fairly easy, since he is the only one who has the job of writing prescriptions.) The fact that each discipline has specific functions led to the need to explore the basic model under which the entire team worked. Should it be the medical, public health, or educational model? These issues were not resolved and a mental health model was not proposed, but everyone present felt this debate should be continued.

Summary

In this chapter much discussion focused upon the element of choice concerning who receives treatment in the community mental health center and who gets referred to a quasi member of the mental health team, the public health nurse. The patients referred to the public health nurse were most often chronic patients. The day may come when patients are able to choose who their care giver will be. When that day arrives it would be nice if the patient could make his choice on the basis of knowledge about what each care giver has to offer and not be caught up in competition and sparring among the various groups of mental health workers.

Chapter Six

FROM THE MOUTHS OF PSYCHOLOGISTS

There are five psychologists from a variety of settings on this panel. Two were from psychiatric crisis units, one from a large state hospital which used therapeutic community concepts, and one from the state's community mental health planning division. The psychologists had strong ideas and opinions, which they expressed openly.

Psychiatric nurses and psychologists have had an interesting history together since the arrival of the clinical psychologist on the psychiatric scene. Brackbill has described this well. Prior to the arrival of the clinical psychologist, doctors and nurses in psychiatric hospitals had a very well prescribed routine. The nurse "ran the ward" and the doctor did the "therapy," wrote orders, prescribed medication and retired to his office. With the arrival of the clinical psychologist, who had a different set of skills, a batch of tests, and endless research projects, the equilibrium was upset. According to Brackbill, mutual suspicion and distrust reigned supreme.[1] We were interested in finding out if the stereotypes the nurse had of the psychologist and the psychologist of the nurse would come out in the panel discussion. As it turned out, the psychologists expressed many ideas about nurses and nursing, women, and their own profession. In this chapter, something of what makes psychologists tick is revealed as well as what they thought made nurses tick. How they viewed the role of the nurse in community mental health is also brought out. The underlying question the psychologists had to ask themselves was, is the nurse a necessary member of the outpatient community mental health center team? It must have been an unnerving thought, particularly with five nurses sitting opposite them who quite obviously thought the nurse was an essential member. However, despite the unnerving effect of the Task Force the psychologists charged forward boldly.

Instead of a lamp—a mop

The first discussant, who was a former member of a family crisis team, took care of the questionnaire in short order by saying that the areas of outpatient care, aftercare services, consultation, and emergency services were part of any crisis service. He then discussed the role of the nurse in that context. He further narrowed his comments by stating that in actuality there

---

[1] Brackbill, G. A.: Psychologists and nurses in the mental hospital, Journal of Psychiatric Nursing, Sept.-Oct. 1967, pp. 432–441.

was a great deal of role blurring on the team* with which he had worked. His feeling about role blurring was that it inspires a sense of sharing, hence satisfaction among team members. He stated that all three of the full-time team members—a psychiatrist, social worker, and nurse—were interchangeable in the treatment of patients. In this setting, patients and their families were assigned to whichever two team members were available or, occasionally, to whomever preferred to work with a particular case. He included evaluation, family treatment, decisions about the therapy schedule, home visits, and the suggesting of medication as shared functions. (The thought in the authors' minds was, "Great Scott, nurses can't even claim knowledge of medication anymore; another sacred cow has bit the dust!") About the area of medication, the discussant said, "I think that after the first year all three of the full-time clinical members acquired a good experience using the psychoactive drugs and simply suggested to the psychiatrist the drug he should prescribe." Traditionally, prescription of medication was an area of expertise reserved for the doctor. However, the nurse also has knowledge of and responsibility for medication. Now it seems the psychiatrist and nurse are sharing this area with social workers and psychologists.

Knowing about and contacting appropriate agencies for longer term care was also shared in equal parts by the psychiatrist, social worker, and nurse on this team. This is an area the nurse and social worker often vie for as their forte. Another shared function in this crisis service was that of home-visiting, which was an important part of the treatment. In this case, too, all functions were shared, but initially the nurse, who had a background of experience in public health nursing, led the way. To the nurse, home-visiting was literally "home ground"; to the other professionals, it was, for a while, foreign land into which they did not venture without the nurse.

This psychologist then discussed areas of specialization, two of which applied particularly to the nurse. There was the matter of giving shots, which the social worker and psychologist were not allowed by law to do, and there was the aspect of being a woman. In his statement about specialization of the nurse, the psychologist commented on some of the positive and negative aspects of the female role. The fact that the nurse was a woman made housework her specialty; this, for some, may have a negative connotation. However, in actual practice it was a valuable and rewarding role. For instance, if one of the patient's problems was the matter of doing domestic chores, the nurse would go into the home and work with the woman giving her courage and support or helping her devise a schedule so that the load did not seem overwhelming. It is axiomatic that the way in which a task is viewed by other members of the team has a great deal to do with how the nurse views it. In

---

* This team is described by Langsley, D., and Kaplan, D., and others: The treatment of families in crisis, New York, 1968, Grune & Stratton, Inc.

this case, the task of organizing housework was seen as practical, valuable, and necessary, and the nurse was the best person on the team to undertake it. It also appeared from the psychologist's comments that the fact that the nurse was a woman was a positive factor in establishing rapport with certain kinds of patients, such as adolescent girls and the shyer, more withdrawn patients. In many respects, he was saying that nurses can capitalize on their feminine role to bring a necessary component to the treatment team. However, if the nurse's claim to uniqueness or if her *raison d'etre* is that she is a woman and can give shots, then we are all treading on pretty thin ice. That isn't much upon which a unique role may be based.

A notable omission in this psychologist's remarks was any reference to the nurse's role in research. One reason for this omission might be that this psychologist's primary task on the team was that of research. We are speculating, but it seems probable that he did not consider the nurse prepared in the area of research, nor perhaps did the nurse. It is also possible that he did not consider the other two professionals prepared in the area either. Unfortunately, this point was not pursued in the later dialogue between the Task Force and the panel members. To summarize this discussant's remarks, it seems fair to say that he was trying very hard to be nice to the group and to affirm that there was, in fact, a unique role for the nurse on an outpatient crisis service in a mental health center, but in reality it would seem he was not too convinced.

Advanced education for nurses? Horrors!

The next psychologist began his remarks by discussing one of his pet peeves, that of the status differences between academicians and the clinicians within a profession. He spoke partly in reference to psychologists and partly in reference to the profession of nursing. He said that there has been a long course of dissension with the academicians detesting the clinicians. In this war of words, the clinicians claim the academicians live in an ivory tower and don't know what is really important and relevant, and the academicians say the clinicians are some form of charlatan practicing on intuition without much cerebration. The psychologist then looked around, saying that things like that aren't supposed to be said and, "We don't have any professors here [besides me], do we?" He then went on to say that he felt the same dissension was present in the nursing profession. The psychologist's guess that this same dissension reigns in the kingdom of nursing as well as the kingdom of psychology is certainly true, as will be noted in Chapters 7 and 8.

This psychologist then dispensed with the format of the Task Force's questionnaire with even greater swiftness than the first by saying that he felt the role of the nurse in any of the five basic components of the community mental health center was defined entirely by her competence. In explaining his statement, he said that he didn't feel therapy was anyone's exclusive bailiwick. It would seem to the authors, however, that he did consider the nurse a new-comer to the therapy scene, which is perhaps true. Nurses have not considered themselves full-fledged psychotherapists until recently. They have taken great care to define "nursing therapy" as opposed to "real therapy," just as they have taken great care to differentiate between "nursing diagnosis" and "real diagnosis." Within the hospital setting in particular, there is a difference between the kinds of problems the nurse usually identifies and does something about and those the doctor identifies and does something about, but the nurse and doctor use many of the same bits of knowledge, and diagnosis is the name of the game. In the area of psychiatry, there is less distinction between the diagnosis a nurse or another professional makes and that which the psychiatrist makes.

This psychologist stated that he saw no limit for the nurse in terms of role. He felt the nurse could venture into areas such as behavior modification and joint family therapy without formal training. "So what if she hasn't had formal training in these areas. All she has to do is get some supervision." He then focused his remarks on what he thought was unique in the role of the nurse. He said that one thing the nurse has that none of the other professionals have is a kind of *unique relationship with the poor*. He substantiated this statement by saying that the nurse has not been a distant professional but has gone into the community and has worked in people's homes. The prototype for this role is, of course, the public health nurse. Historically, the mental health nurse in the community mental health center may owe more to the public health nurse than she realizes at this point. It may well be that the public health nurse has paved the way for the inclusion of the nurse on the community mental health center outpatient team. The psychologist made an interesting point by comparing the nurse's mobility in the community to other professions, saying that anyone else who leaves the office is questioned and is often accused of trying to establish a counter-trend or of behaving inappropriately. Without identifying *it*, the psychologist said that the nurse has something in terms of her image, unique to the profession of nursing. "It" seemed to be something in her background, training, and experience *that none of the other professionals have*, and part of this "it" was mobility and acceptance by the community and the poor. This image in the community may be an important factor and something nurses need to identify and maintain. However, at this point one of the members of the Task Force quipped that perhaps nurses' closeness with the poor had something to do with their own place on the salary scale. It is a thought.

The psychologist-professor next focused on the question of whether additional preparation was necessary for the nurse who worked in the community mental health center. He stated quite emphatically that he did not consider additional *formal* training necessary. His position was predicated on his opinion that nurses are unique and that this uniqueness might be destroyed by additional preparation. He said, "I think we have discovered historically that as you increase the years people go to school, you raise their degree, which may be a necessary prerequisite for the job. However, what you get, really, is some improvement of skills, which is minimal compared to the change in professional status. That is the issue, it seems to me. You don't get better professionals; if anything, you get people who suddenly start looking down on certain kinds of work and begin to change their role. You start eliminating service people and start developing administrative people, grant getters, and journal authors." He continued by saying that he felt strongly that additional preparation could dilute and change the image of the nurse to the extent that the nurse's unique image with certain segments of the population would be lost. The authors do not agree with the discussant in toto, but it does seem that he makes some sound points and raises some interesting questions.

In pursuing the line of thought about the questionable value of advanced preparation for nurses, he remarked that what happens when persons become "professional" is that they start talking a lot of jargon: "If you use the right terminology and jargon, you're in." It is very interesting that just as he, a psychologist, was downgrading the use of jargon, the social workers had praised it. This does seem to be an example of the kind of intellectual snobbery that exists among psychiatric professionals concerning the issue of psychiatric terminology. But, we ask, why fight it? Granted, knowledge of terminology is a questionable yardstick by which to judge a professional's competence, but in reality it may be important for nurses to know the terminology in order to be accepted by other psychiatric professionals. Does knowing psychiatric terminology, psychiatric diagnostic categories and psychoanalytic theory make a nurse less a nurse? The psychologist cautioned nurses in the use of psychiatric knowledge, however. The jargon and traditional diagnostic categories form a structure that may work to the detriment of the patient. It is a well-accepted fact that once a patient is labeled a character disorder, for example, he or she is regarded as hopeless. A far more helpful approach would be to work on a problem-solving basis, which, this discussant remarked, nurses are more likely to do. Perhaps this is an area at which nurses, along with other professionals in community mental health, need to take a more careful look. It is interesting that one of the consistent things nurses have said about themselves as well as a characteristic identified by other professionals is that of practicality. There seems to be a consensus among the professionals interviewed by the Task Force that the nurse is a pragmatist. This practical orientation is a valuable characteristic and may make the nurse's approach to patients different from that of other professionals. Perhaps the problem-solving approach to psychiatric problems is a tool that nurses have which they can bring to the community mental health center team and, in addition, teach to others.

This psychologist summarized his remarks by saying that the nurse needed, in his opinion, basic nursing education as well as a broad, well-integrated liberal arts background. Preparation beyond the basic level, except for on-the-job learning, he felt was useless. He identified a key problem, in his closing remarks—that the nurse frequently does not take the initiative. He characterized this lack of initiative as an "I'd better wait for the doctor's order" tendency. Nurses are "raised" in a hospital which is a hierarchical institution, he said, and it may be that this training is a mixed blessing; it accounts, on the one hand, for a uniqueness in the nursing role and for part of her public image, and, on the other, for her fear of taking the initiative in decision-making. This discussant ended his remarks in much the same vein as the first had by saying that nurses may have some unique experience and knowledge that none of the other professionals have but without being sure what "it" was. The question, again left unanswered, was, is the nurse really a necessary member of the outpatient community mental health center team?

The "it" factor

"Let's blur the role of the nurse, which means nurses should not go around acting like nurses," was the opening remark of the next discussant. He took issue with the two previous discussants who had said that role blurring should be employed by community mental health center teams. This discussant proposed, in contrast to role blurring or role expansion (which are current clichés) a role sharpening. He said that the role of nurses will be shaped a great deal by the kind of setting in which they operate. In an inpatient setting that is based on milieu therapy concepts, the role of the nurse will be that of milieu therapist. In a setting that is devoted to individual psychotherapy, the role of the nurse may be quite different. The discussant did not say, interestingly enough, that in an individual therapy oriented setting the role of the nurse would become that of psychotherapist. He said the role would be "quite different." The role of the nurse in that kind of setting is indeed quite different. The nurse in that setting, in our experience, is primarily custodial. The doctor-patient relationship is the end-all and be-all of therapy, and the prevailing attitude of the doctor in that setting is that the nurse will not harm the patient. Rarely is she seen as a potential therapist. In the hospitals of this type that do promote individual nurse-patient relationships, it is frequently at the insistence of the nurse and then under the doctor's close supervision. The nurse is not viewed as a therapist competent in her own right.

However, despite this discussant's slip regarding the nurse as a therapist, for which the committee will forgive him, he went on to make some important statements about role sharpening with regard to the nurse. He said that he would like to see the preparation in basic nursing strengthened, not just the basic nursing skills, but the attitudes of the nurse. For him the image of a nurse conjured up certain kinds of attitudes, *a concern about patients that is somewhat different from the kind of concern that other professionals have.* A kind of "it" factor? He felt the nurse functioned with a degree of closeness and intimacy with patients not tolerated by other professionals. In terms of caring for basic needs of patients, he felt the nurse was more comfortable and competent than any of the other professionals. This discussant felt that many patients' feeling of rapport with the nurse have to do with her ability to deal with intimate basic functions that may concern the patient. He felt that the image and major role of the nurse is to ease pain. He differentiated the patient's image in this way: "The doctor may cure me, the social worker may help me figure out where to go to get a welfare check, but if I'm hurting I call for the nurse."

He went on to emphasize that he agreed with the first discussant in that nurses need not emulate the other professions nor try to talk their language. He said that in his experience, on any treatment team regardless of size, the psychologist was the most likely person to ask "why"; that is, why did the patient develop this pathology as opposed to some other form of psychopathology, why does the patient act one way instead of another? He said: "I would not like to see the nurse give up her tradition, emulate the psychologist, and try to beat him to the punch to say 'Why'." There is a difference in background, this discussant went on to say, that makes the nurse different than the psychologist. He did not identify the differences in background between nurses and psychologists, but they seem obvious. The liberal arts and science base of the nurse and psychologist is probably similar, but whereas the nurse is "raised" in a hospital, the psychologist is "raised" in a lab full of rats. He felt that nurses should be more assertive in getting other members of the team to look at the present and how people are hurting. He said that he would like to see the nurse bring the other professionals back to earth and insert her point of view. The nursing point of view is important and needs to be inserted and emphasized on any team of the community mental health center, whether it be inpatient, emergency, or outpatient. The nurse is concerned with people's hurt and their present situation.

The natural superiority of women

One obviously important factor in the role of the nurse had, at this point, been overlooked—the fact that most nurses are women. The next discussant, a clinical psychologist, focused on this issue. "For one thing," he said, "I think the nurse offers again and again a feminine outlook which is unique; although even with all our research we psychologists can't specify or spell it out." "Women should not fight for equality with men, as a French philosopher said, as they will only lose their natural superiority." The authors think this could also be translated to read: nurses should not fight for equality with other members of the community mental health center team or they will lose their natural inferiority. The authors disbelieve the veracity of the French philosopher's statement. It is easy or perhaps soothing to women to say that the woman, although she remains in the background, is superior to the man. However, our society doesn't believe it. An illustration of prevailing attitudes toward women is the following experience of one of the authors. She was attending a meeting of the American Medical Association concerning the issue of therapeutic abortion. After listening to the arguments pro and con, she gathered her courage and proposed to the group of doctors, all male, that a board of three women review and pass judgment on all males requesting a vasectomy just as a board of three men reviews and passes judgment on all women requesting a therapeutic abortion or tubal ligation. The looks of shock and the nervous laughter that followed this proposal were quite revealing and said something important about the real place of women in our society. The men clearly could not imagine such a role for women but took the same role as a matter of course for themselves.

Now all this is not to say that there is not something unique about the feminine viewpoint and that this is not valuable. Further, the feminine viewpoint is something a team can ill-afford to lack. Since the majority of nurses are women, planners of community mental health center teams would be well advised to consider including the nurse on this basis as well as for her professional orientation to the patient. As the clinical psychologist stated, the nurse offers again and again, perhaps more by chance than design, a feminine outlook which is unique. He ruefully said again that what precisely is unique about the feminine outlook is something psychologists have been unable to identify.

The clinical psychologist also said that nurses must do something to change the image of the nurse from bedpan carrier to that of an independent professional. He suggested that one of the ways to change this image was to begin with the nurses' education and thereby inculcate a new attitude in them. The attitudes instilled by the educational system, as the clinical psychologist pointed out, are very important. However, the other side of the coin is the expectations of the nurse in the work setting. In some institutional settings, nurses are not permitted to function as other than doctors' assistants. A study conducted in 1968 by Harrington and Theis demonstrated this quite well. Baccalaureate graduates employed as staff nurses in three hospitals were interviewed regarding their ability to practice what they, the interviewees, regarded as professional nursing functions. Nurses from the two "typical" hospitals revealed that they were constrained in their attempts to relate to the total needs of the patient by the expectations of administrative personnel, by the method of functional assignments, by the assignment of nonnursing functions, and by hierarchical ladder-like channels of communication. In the institutional setting where nurses were expected and permitted to attend to the total needs of the patient including extensive discharge planning, there was respect for the nurses' judgment from other collaborating staff, including the physicians.[2] So, while the attitudes instilled as part of nursing education have received a certain

---

[2] Harrington, H., and Theis, E. C.: Institutional factors perceived by baccalaureate graduates as influencing their performance as staff nurses, Nursing Research **17**(3):228–235, May-June 1968.

amount of fire in this book, the expectations of the institution must also be considered, as it may be that institutions destroy attitudes which the schools have built. Perhaps it is in keeping with the fact that institutional factors influence the functioning of the nurse that the psychologist stated his belief that psychiatric nurses were leading the way in dispensing with the "hand-maiden to the doctor" image and creating a role for themselves as independent practitioners. It is difficult to determine how much of this increased professionalism is due to the personalities and education of psychiatric nurses and how much is attributable to expectations in the work setting. In previous years, particularly prior to the implementation of Maxwell Jones' concepts of therapeutic communities[3] (he felt nurses and their assistants played a key role), the psychiatric nurse's role was to provide custodial care only. Since the advent of newer concepts of psychiatric care, it does seem that the psychiatric nurse's role has undergone change. This change toward greater independence as a therapeutic agent and a professional may also have to do with the greater tendency for psychiatrists to distribute power. This distribution has been suggested by one writer as being particularly prevalent in the community mental health setting and as having a great deal to do with the tendency for nurses with a master's degree to enter the community mental health field.[4] All things considered, however, it is still an uphill battle for most nurses to establish themselves as independent practitioners. The experiences of the members of the Task Force suggest that it is easier for the nurse to establish herself as an independent professional in the community mental health field, but this again depends upon the philosophy of the director of the mental health center. The circle can be vicious or delightful. On the one hand the centers may give little recognition or opportunity for professional performance, in which case they stifle initiative and finally fail to attract interested, well-qualified professional nurses. On the other hand, just the opposite can occur when recognition and opportunity are given, thus stimulating and attracting other enthusiastic, well-qualified professional nurses.

In suggesting to nurses that they take steps to change their image, the clinical psychologist said that psychologists have tried many avenues to change their image such as the use of public relations firms and lobbyists. He did not specify what psychologists dislike about their own image, but it may well be the image of the man who is immersed in a battery of tests from which he derives magical, dynamic formulations and who is uncommonly bound up in basic research as the only path to true knowledge. He did say that psychologists have not arrived at any set of acceptable solutions to the problem and that, therefore, nurses would have to find their own way.

---

[3] Jones, M.: The therapeutic community, New York, 1953, Basic Books.
[4] Christman, L.: Nurse-physician communication, Journal of the American Medical Association **194**(5):151–156, 1965.

Nurses must define their role or others will do it for them

The next discussant opened his remarks by observing that, with all due respect to his colleagues and the Task Force, there certainly was a great deal of eagerness to tell nurses what their role should be but that the Task Force had set itself up for this by inviting the psychologists to talk. His point was well stated; however, to reiterate, the goal of the Task Force in asking other professionals what they thought the role of the nurse should be was (1) to find out what others thought and felt as necessary information to define the role of the nurse, (2) to shake their stereotypes a little and do some educating of the panelists, and (3) to persuade professionals to think about *nurses* as members of the community mental health center in the same way psychiatrists, psychologists and social workers are thought of as members. Again, however, he made a cogent point; that is, if nurses don't define their role for themselves, and in a hurry, the very eagerness of other professionals to define roles and the pressing staffing problems of community mental health will define it for them. The authors are inclined to think that this process might very well happen and that nurses could find themselves out in the cold. Everybody agrees that nurses have a role on inpatient services (somebody must take care of the patient), but there is no such general consensus regarding her role in the four other essential components of the community mental health center. Unless nurses stand up and shout, define what they can do in other settings, and sell their viewpoint as valuable, nurses will be farmed out to inpatient services only.

This psychologist made another reasonable point when he said that there is such diversity in settings and such complexity in the community mental health movement, whatever definition of role nurses come to, it must be flexible. This statement should not be taken to mean that the nurse must be all things to all people—too many nurses already think that—but that the role of the nurse must encompass diversity of function.

This discussant's particular frustration was the lack of a scientific basis for manpower utilization. He said that there is no theory to guide us toward an intelligent rationale for utilization of existing manpower. The result is a system of community mental health that has grown like Topsy. First the physician came as captain of the team and gradually other people were added as arms of the physician. The system grew without a scientific base whereby different functions could be assigned to different people based on different kinds of training. He continued by saying, "This is not to say that there have not been studies, but they seem to me to be backwards because they go find somebody who is already doing a job, take voluminous notes and do a factor analysis comparing his job to somebody else's and whatever is left over is considered unique." He felt that members of a profession should be able to look at a situation and know approximately what they can do before they are called upon to function. Once the professional is in the situation he might take on new and different responsibilities. These new skills could then be recycled back to the educational programs. Basically, the psychologist was saying that nothing need remain static; the closed system is a short-lived system. Relevant to the point of trying to find a balance between having a well-identified role and yet remaining open to try new areas was this discussant's statement and plea that nurses not be afraid to push into new areas. "Any professional worth his salt begins to push the boundaries and when he does this he starts growing as a real 'pro'."

The discussion then moved on to whether or not additional preparation was necessary for the nurse in community mental health centers. This discussant expressed the feeling that graduate school above all else teaches the student to use judgment and instills a feeling of self-confidence. He stated, "The essence of being professional is using judgment." It seems that judgment and self-confidence may be indirect products of graduate school. "Nobody takes a course called Judgment 101 or Self-Confidence 102, but they are unmistakably there in most people at the conclusion of graduate education." He said that graduate education was necessary for the nurse in certain areas of community mental health, although he did not specify the areas that he thought required graduate education.

Summary

The panel discussion ended and frequently sharp dialogue between the Task Force and the panel of psychologists began. The points focused on by the Task Force were the questions of role sharpening versus role blurring. One of the nurses was quite defensive. She had heard the panel saying the nurse can have what's left after all the other professions have defined their role. This defensiveness seems to be common among nurses at this point, perhaps because for so long it has been true. The nurse has been and still is considered less a professional than the doctor or psychologist.

The opinions stated by the psychologists regarding the lack of need for graduate education also came in for sharp review by the Task Force. It was pointed out that it was quite incongruous for the psychologist with a Ph.D. to negate graduate education for nurses. The Task Force did not "buy" this note of anti-intellectualism.

Chapter Seven

MULTIDISCIPLINARY POTPOURRI

The decision to meet with representatives of all the disciplines with whom we had previously talked was based on curiosity more than the expectation of new data. However, we were pleased on both counts. We had the opportunity, though brief, to observe how a group of strangers, who knew little more about each other than their mental health titles, related and solved the problem presented to them. The questions given them were identical to the ones presented to the homogenous discipline groupings.

The multidiscipline group was composed of a psychiatric technician with long experience in a state-operated mental health center who was known for her intellectual ability and her willingness to participate in theoretical discussions; a nurse educator and teacher of psychiatric nursing who enjoyed talking about roles; a psychologist who had written about nurse role in the emergency psychiatric service of a mental health center; a social worker who had recently been involved in the planning and implementing of a new community mental health center and had also worked with the nursing discipline; and a psychiatrist and author who was opinionated about mental health centers generally, and nursing particularly.

The last shall be first—the first shall be last

The discussion began with the nurse educator leading off, as was her choice. She apparently felt she had to or the discussion would not get "off the ground." Her beginning sentence was, "I would like to start first, and it is about determining the role of the nurse that I wish to speak, which will provide an opportunity for the others to respond." Her following statements lent credence to the premise for this book in that she said, "I believe the interdiscipline context is going to be the crucial baseline on which we can begin to differentiate what the roles are and to look at the similarities and differences." She then proceeded to identify the following as roles and abilities of nurses:

1. The nurse's ability to create and maintain the therapeutic milieu
2. The role of the nurse in family therapy in the home setting
3. The nurse's ability to immediately assess the patient's mental and physical health problems
4. The nurse's role in the initial intervention process, such as, relieving of stress in the patient and his family
5. The nurse's ability to synthesize knowledge from many varying fields to give her a broadened perspective to look into the patient's problem

6. The nurse's proximity to the patient, as well as the nurse's ease of movement in the territory of the home or hospital
7. The flexibility of the nurse in spite of all the other people saying how rigid she is
8. The nurse's role in coordinating patient care
9. The broad life experience that the nurse offers the patient based upon her experiences with varying kinds of patients in a variety of stressful situations

The psychiatrist followed this presentation and spoke from the point of view of the "consumer of nurses or an employer—someone who hires nurses." In his usual witty style, he stated, "I can't say I use them because I used to say that until a nurse friend pointed out that that was a very bad word for nurses." He was, of course, referring to the word "use." The psychiatrist, while listening to the previous discussion, found himself asking about the attributes of nurses. He organized them into categories and presented them for all of us to hear and ponder. They were:

Technical attributes of nurses

1. The specific act of "administering drugs and the reality that even though we don't talk about it, most patients in community health programs take drugs at some point in their treatment."
2. The nurse is a member of the only discipline that characteristically has experience supervising nonprofessionals and that experience ranges from minimal to quite extensive. None of the other disciplines has any predictable experience along these lines.
3. A nurse is trained ("at least this year") in care-oriented institutions. This is different from other disciplines.
4. The nurse is the only person who has any experience in the management of the wards and who can predictably handle that responsibility.
5. Public health experience or training, which includes a very important aspect of community work, such as home evaluation and family-oriented counseling.

Personal attributes of nurses

1. Nurses tend to be pragmatic.
2. Nurses tend to be task-oriented both by inclination and conditioning.
3. Nurses tend to have a very high perseverence level and a high frustration tolerance. The psychiatrist's comments about this are worthy of a quote: "They complain a hell of a lot, but they persevere, and they have the highest perseverence level of any of the mental health disciplines as an overall generalization. Mental health people are terrible quitters, you know; they are like itinerant laborers who move around all the time because they can't cope with things, and nurses stick things out, and that's barring pregnancy, marriage, and all that."

4. Nurses are intelligent even though they tend to be cowed by intellectual types.
5. Nurses are orderly even if they keep trying to outgrow it and deny it. The rest of the mental health field is disorderly, and the nurse lends some stability to this disorder.

Experiential attributes of nurses

1. Nursing is the only profession with the exception of psychiatry that has predictably had hospital experience.
2. Nurses have had a lot of experience working with doctors. They have coped before with a medically oriented power structure and are not as apt to want to destroy the authority of the psychiatrists as are the other disciplines. In a multidisciplinary team where the psychiatrist team leader is being shaken and threatened by the other disciplines, he can usually rely upon the nurse for support. Nurses may tear the psychiatrist down when talking to other nurses, but for some reason, she projects a degree of loyalty to the physician on the multidisciplinary team. (The Task Force wonders if this may be a manipulation game on the part of the nurse or an unconscious adherence to the Florence Nightingale pledge.)

An experiential disadvantage, which the psychiatrist identified as the main disadvantage, was nurses' "having been trained in a rigid hierarchy that has limited their ability to comfortably assume attributes of freedom and to work in a multidisciplinary setting." He blamed the "unisexual rigid hierarchy authoritarian system" of nursing for this. Be it loyalty, agreement, or manipulation, the Task Force has no argument with this stated disadvantage.

Nurses function in all five components of the mental health center in this particular psychiatrist's domain. He saw problems in the areas of skilled consultation, but he also saw the other disciplines as having the same problems. He felt that nurses were not as involved in consultation, education, and research and that areas of expansion in these roles should be in relation to inpatient and outpatient centers.

Good old fashioned competence

The social worker began by talking about who was and who was not prepared to work in comprehensive mental health centers. "I think we all probably agree that none of the disciplines, I am speaking for social workers at least, are really prepared for community mental health work as such." He agreed with the psychiatrist that the nurse is more flexible in terms of traditionally being where the action is. The social worker called upon the public health nursing model to best describe the positive functioning of the nurse. He also invoked Gerald Caplan, who had said in a seminar on mental health consultation that the most gifted mental health consultant Dr. Caplan knew was a psychiatric nurse. "Of course," said the social worker, "what he was talking about was good old fashioned competence. I think the field is open to all comers, and the competence of the nurse has been well established." He did not define competence, but said he would like to see nursing "a bit more aggressive." He did not see the nurse as being already prepared with skills. The social worker then ended his part of the commentary by saying that he hoped the psychiatric nurse would challenge the "ingrown traits" of the Triumvirate and pick up the things that they were "missing." He did not elaborate on what these traits were.

Behavior change is the name of the game

The psychologist spoke next and said he saw the nurse's amount of patient contact as placing her in a unique position. This position can be viewed positively and negatively. "I think behavior change is the name of the game, and the nurse's role, traditionally, perhaps has been one of maintenance of behaviors and not one of how you bring about behavior change and the necessary bunch of skills that go along with that." He used the inpatient setting to develop this point and observed that it has been nursing and nursing personnel who had encouraged good patient adjustment to the ward. He questioned, as indeed he should, whether this was an important behavior change, or was it not more useful to encourage adjustment for behavior change after hospitalization, which he felt was less used as a medium for learning experiences by nurses. "So I would see one thing as being necessary here [for the nurse], and that is a firmer grounding in personality dynamics, learning theory and again, really in general, an understanding of behavior—why people act as they do, how you can intervene in the pattern of behavior and change them significantly." He cited warmth, nurturance, and maternal feelings, supposedly characteristic of the nurse, as tending to fix and reinforce behaviors that were not effective. He felt that warmth was necessary, but declared that if it was not used correctly it would reinforce maladaptive behavior. This echos the nurse clinicians' concept of educated use of caring as discussed in Chapter 8.

In listening to the members of the other disciplines present their views, he came up with the idea that psychiatric nurses should develop consulting relationships "with school nurses, public health nurses, and others who see potential patients for the first time." This had apparently not occurred to him before, a phenomenon which was not unusual in the groups we had interviewed. He began to develop a framework for the nurse in the community mental health center to become involved in preventive psychiatry. He believed that the emergency room setting was a good place for the nurse to be and made some astute observations to consider the involvement of psychiatric nurses in research. They bear quoting, particularly since they come from a member of a profession whose "pure" research has been a point of envy of some. "As far as research goes, I think that the nurse being found in so many different settings offers a unique opportunity for her to do some down-to-earth research. The journals are filled with studies which are interesting from an academic point of view but have very little relationship to what is actually going on. For these reasons, the nurse is in a good position to possibly conduct some realistic studies and to apply some of the research found in the journals but which never gets down to the actual working situation."

The last person to speak, as was her choice, was the psychiatric technician who said that the panel had started out with a nurse and ended with a technician which she felt was appropriate, since the psychiatric technicians were under nursing direction. She said that she saw the nurse and technician roles similarly, particularly in regard to their closeness to the patients. She talked about the nurse's involvement with daily living experiences and patient teaching. She saw the nurse as the coordinator in assisting patients, not only in inpatient settings, but in transitional and outpatient settings. She stressed community work with parent-teacher associations, women's groups, schools, and the courts. She hoped she wasn't stepping on social work's toes by seeing the nurse as helpful in researching the community and making the appropriate referral. She said that she was reluctant to reiterate what the other disciplines had said, but did not recall that any one had mentioned the mountains of paper work that nurses do in the psychiatric settings. No one had mentioned anything about that "functional" part of the nurse's role.

How and where does one learn consultation

A joint discussion followed in which consultation was the initial topic. The nurse educator explained the lack of master's level preparation for consultation by stating that schools are leaning toward this subject in post-master's education. The social worker cited the same shortcoming in schools of social work. The psychiatrist pointed out that nurses do indeed consult in pre- and postnatal situations and other crisis areas whether or not there is formal education in this area. The public health nurse could use the input of the psychiatric nurse to enhance her understanding of these crucial areas.

The topic of consultation led to a discussion of the need to learn more about the community, not only for nursing but for all disciplines. The nurse educator said, "We're too much hospital oriented. I'm not saying that we want all of it discontinued, but I think we need to think more about a community orientation. The dynamics within a hospital structure are quite different from those of a community." The social worker agreed and said, "It is only in the past few years that there has been such a tremendous interest in community organization and social action on the part of social workers and this is the result of a lot of feeling that the social worker has forgotten his advocate role—his role of organizing the disadvantaged and the minority persons. Social work may be in the process of rediscovering its social conscience." He wondered if nursing had yet arrived at this point in order to "move out" in a social action sense. The social worker felt, as did most other disciplines involved, that perhaps the nurses need to be more aggressive and outspoken. He felt that nursing needs to know something about power and politics as a means "of bringing about change not only in terms of the community but in terms of their own organization." He also implied that nurses need this knowledge to work with other disciplines.

A mental health center is not what it says it is

Training, and for what, was the next subject. The psychiatrist stated, "Our patients are at times more sophisticated than we are and they recognize that a mental health center is really a mental illness center. If you look around nationally at what is being done in mental health centers, you find that they are treating emotionally disturbed people. They are in fact a new kind of treatment facility, lodged differently institutionally with their resources deployed a little differently, but they are treating ill people, nonetheless." He said that mental health people utilize ninety percent of their time in talking about the wonderful things they are going to do and ten percent in actually doing it. He felt quite strongly that as yet there is no evidence that we know much about the preventive aspects of mental illness. "I would like to think that it will show, but until we have some more defensible demonstrations of this, I think that what we really need is to have our mental illness service functioning well in all communities, and this requires more manpower."

What's going to happen to the children?

Quite naturally, from the discussion of lack of knowledge regarding prevention, came the topic of the future expansion in treatment services for psychiatrically ill children. The psychiatrist pointed the finger at all mental health professionals, saying that we dodge the issue of the ill child and treat "nail biters and bedwetters, and let the juvenile court system handle all the rest—those who end up in the state hospital." Nursing is also lax in this field with too few programs offering preparation in child psychiatry. The psychiatrist predicted that the recent joint commission[1] for the study of children should give impetus to more treatment programs for children.

Tuning out what's not nice

Another area in which mental health people are unprepared is the treatment of that "whole spectrum of behaviors that are currently considered bad, immoral, or evil. They are now subject to a social control system." The psychiatrist further predicted that persons who exhibit poor behavior patterns

---

[1] Joint Commission on Mental Health of Children: Crisis in child mental health; challenge for the 70's, New York, 1970, Harper & Row, Publishers.

such as alcoholism, drug addiction, and juvenile delinquency are going to "move into the mental health system over the dead bodies of most of the people now observed in leadership positions in mental health facilities. None of the professionals recognize this in the training programs, and none of them really have adjusted themselves as to how to turn out the people to handle this problem." No one in the room challenged the psychiatrist's predictions. In fact, heads nodded in agreement. He went on further to predict the obsolescence of the public mental health center and saw the mental health center replaced by small multidisciplinary private practices. Professionals then will be judged on their productivity in the course of a work week. Woe be it, then, to those who work ten percent and dream ninety percent. Nurses, along with the members of other disciplines, will need to be prepared to work in these settings.

The intellectuals versus the earthy types

All the nurses present agreed and again alluded to the deficits in the current educational system for nursing in undergraduate and graduate schools, where the psychopath model and the intrapsychic model are taught instead of the far more relevant issues of social process. Poverty and affluence and their influence on child rearing were given as examples. Nursing education's current gap with clinical practice was seen as the reason why so many undergraduate and graduate programs stand on the traditional psychiatric models. "The key deficit in nursing education is that so many nurse educators quit practicing when they start teaching, and this builds in obsolescence for nursing education," said the psychiatrist. The nurse educator on the panel defended this practice saying, "The problem is in the schools and is the result of heavy teaching loads all instructors carry." The psychiatrist suggested that the schools should staff their programs on the assumption that every semester a designated number of faculty would be away doing clinical work or something similar. One of the Task Force suggested that clinical specialists in the community could be used to enrich faculty with what is current and pertinent. This suggestion for a two-way street prompted the nurse educator to mention a concern she has long had, "a trend toward anti-intellectualism developing within the nursing field." She spoke of attending meetings in which there was a division with one faction so down to earth that they were unable or unwilling to deal with an idea or theory. She believed this division would be perpetuated unless we really brought both in balance by bringing the field and academic roles closer together. It is interesting to note that she chose not to or was unable to deal with the suggestion of bringing clinical people in as faculty, but instead dealt with the fear of an anti-intellectual trend [being perpetuated by those in clinical practice]. (At this point an area of fruitful discussion for this group or a group of nurses might have been a theoretical one based on the reasons for this anti-intellectual trend which has frightened some nurse academicians. One cannot help but ponder which occurred first—the anti-intellectual movement or the so-called intellectuals moving away from the "down to earth" area of clinical practice. There seems to be little problem from the viewpoint of clinical practice in bringing into one's setting the university faculty, but one perceives some difficulty when the situation is reversed. Some clinicians with whom the Task Force has talked have the notion that they are on display or the university is doing them a favor when they ask them to teach a class, or, worse yet, that as clinicians they might contaminate the environment of students. This trend, the Task Force believes, in all fairness, is changing with the help of the people in the academic setting who have initiated frequent joint meetings where colleague status is encouraged. When this occurs and when we can pool knowledge and work together utilizing experience and education, we believe we will be less caught up in worries about the polarization of intellect.)

Another factor that may affect clinical practice and the academic milieu is the economic one. The psychiatrist pointed out that in medicine the neurotic balance has been maintained because the educator in medical schools has the prestige and the practitioner receives the ample financial rewards. This, he suggested, was not a bad balance if you must divide it. Nursing, on the other hand, falls short, because it does not balance out. The educator not only has the most prestige but also the most money. This is an interesting notion and the Task Force cannot help but wonder if the current trend toward higher remuneration for clinical practice has not helped to give clinical practitioners confidence to challenge the occasionally ivory towered nursing academicians.

What's a nurse, Mommy?

The discussion focused upon the variations in nurse preparation and the confusion that all disciplines, including nursing, have as a result of the varying preparation. No one disputed this. The social worker introduced to the discussion "the very fact that some of the old status differences are breaking down." He wondered whether we should be concerned with various hierarchies in educational preparation, since there is "increasing emphasis on competence regardless of your discipline, regardless of your years of training." The entry of the indigenous worker who is regarded as qualified by life experiences is an instance of this change in the system. "I think we all know people who have not had professional training but who will go out into the field and get the job done. They seem to *feel* what's going on; they organize a group of poor people and get the community behind them, which some of *us* fail to do. They have a natural endowment, a certain kind of empathy. They speak the language of the people with whom they are working. The highly trained professional is at a disadvantage, naturally, in relation to the indigenous worker who speaks the language, who is trusted, and who has natural empathy." This conversation led to the basic question of whether education and training are as important as the person himself. The psychiatrist felt that "competence is measured by the goals of the system in which that person is working," and said, "I find that most systems don't define their goals. Most mental health administrators have a terrible time deciding what kind of people they want to hire because they don't know what they're there to do, and so fall back on formal credentials to decide who to hire. We asked eight mental health centers what the center's job was, and half didn't have any idea, and the rest said, 'do good work'." This very basic question got no further in this discussion, and the fact that it did not makes one wonder if it is an answerable question, or is the issue of credentialed or noncredentialed competence too powerfully laden to be dealt with by professionals subjectively involved?

Summary

This interdisciplinary panel demonstrated that not only can mental health persons talk to each other, but also that they can really disagree. The Task Force found the areas of nurse attributes, behavior change, issues of competency and its deviations, and the issues of intellectual polarization in nursing most provocative. Some of the implications of this discussion provided the basis for the concluding chapters of this book.

PART THREE
Nursing—As We See Ourselves

Chapter Eight

NURSE CLINICIANS— PSYCHIATRIC NURSES TELL IT LIKE IT IS

Those nurses most "in trouble" and about whom this book is written are the nurse clinicians in community mental health centers. The four nurses on this panel were some of the clinicians who are changing the image of nursing. A statement that typified not the consensus of the panel but its spirit was, "The way the word 'caring' is used by the supposed leaders in nursing education just infuriates me." The stereotype of the nurse as a passive-aggressive creature was not portrayed in this discussion. It was a pleasure to listen to their arguments, their frank discussion and disagreement, and to see the aggressiveness with which they tackled the problem of defining the role of the nurse in the community mental health center. From the opening of the discussion to its close one hour later, there was hardly a pause in the lively dialogue. The areas of strongest controversy were: (1) the unique role of the nurse in the community mental health center; (2) the concept of care and, secondarily, cure and coordination; (3) the necessary educational preparation for the nurse in the community mental health center; (4) the place of the nurse in the mental health hierarchy; and (5) the care of the chronically ill patient. The areas of agreement among the clinicians were: (1) that the nurse has a valuable role in all the elements of the community mental health center; (2) the age-old truism that nursing does not convey status or money to its practitioners; (3) the functional roles of the nurse in the community mental health center; (4) the educational preparation for nurses in research; (5) discontent with the traditional role of the nurse as the handmaiden to the doctor; and (6) the X factor. In discussing these areas, they were quick to challenge each other's ideas as well as the traditional role of the nurse. The nurses conveyed competence, intelligence, and aggressiveness. They discussed the issues with considerable humor and demolished the questionnaire in a beautiful sort of way. In this chapter, the areas of controversy will be presented first, then the areas of agreement.

Uniqueness—necessary question or needless hang-up?

The task of defining the unique role of the nurse proved to be difficult for the nurses. Attempts to define uniqueness in terms of what the nurse does led to a temporary dead-end. The discussion was concentrated for some time on the uniqueness of the nurse in the inpatient setting. It soon became clear that attempting to define uniqueness according to the setting and the functions within that setting was not possible. The equation that twenty-four hour care plus administration of medication equals the uniqueness of nurses, does not compute. The equation that caring equals the uniqueness of nurses also does not compute satisfactorily. Adding or substituting the words cure and coordination did not improve the situation. Silence reigned for a short time among the panel, then was broken by the question, "Does it have to be a word?" This question was followed by another, "Do we have to define our uniqueness? Is it really necessary?" And therein lies the crux of the matter. Does the role of the nurse have to be defined by a single word or trilogy of words? Secondly, the question was, "Does uniqueness need to be defined at all?" The arguments for defining the uniqueness of the nurse's role were based, in part, upon the sentiment that if nurses don't define their uniqueness, they are going to be out of a job. That others (doctors, social workers, community mental health workers, and psychiatric technicians) will "take over" was an expression of this sentiment. Many functions of the nurse, it was felt, are being performed by other professionals and nonprofessionals, and this may constitute a threat to the existence of nursing. Consistent with this argument was the statement that nurses had indiscriminately delegated responsibilities to other disciplines, thereby diminishing their profession and giving up something of their uniqueness. This argument is supported by at least one writer who agrees that this delegation of nursing responsibility has been detrimental. "The managerial practice of nursing has the possibility of gradually eroding the clinical practice of nursing."[1] In attempting to resolve the nursing shortage by adopting a managerial model whereby nurses give care through others, the profession has done itself, the patient, and the doctor a disservice. In addition, the implication of this article was that this difference between medicine and nursing in the model of giving care has not only been a detriment to the nursing profession but has created communication problems between physician and nurse as well.[2] The proponents of this argument on the panel concluded that nursing must define its uniqueness to preserve itself as a profession.

The arguments *against* the necessity for defining uniqueness were that there is an ever *decreasing* body of uniqueness in every profession and the profession of nursing need not worry about defining uniqueness. Everyone is sharing functions and responsibilities. The observation was made that no other profession seems quite as worried about its own uniqueness as is the nursing profession.

Another argument *for* defining uniqueness was that it is necessary to avoid being "dumped on" by other disciplines. Medicine, it was felt by the panel, only delegates to nursing what it is no longer interested in doing. Nurses have consistently been anxious to be all things to all people and have been grateful

---

[1] Christman, L.: Nurse-physician communications in the hospital, Journal of the American Medical Association **194**(5): 151, 1965.
[2] *Ibid*, p. 154.

for the opportunity to assume these responsibilities. The failure has not been that nursing has accepted increased responsibility, but that it has not been discriminating in that which it has assumed. Rather than being gifts, some of these new duties have been crumbs, or worse, garbage. Perhaps the importance of defining nursing's uniqueness is so that the individual nurse has a basis for refusing or accepting functions. However, other panel members were less concerned about the "dumping syndrome," and the controversy continued. Some members felt that defining the role of the nurse rigidly would lead to a boring life devoid of challenges and creativity. There was consensus that "dumping" is in the eye of the giver as well as the receiver. A task given over out of respect for competence is likely to be accepted in like manner. However, a task delegated to someone lower in the hierarchy because the task is distasteful is another story. Agreement on the central issue of whether defining uniqueness was necessary was not reached.

Care, cure, and constipation?

The concept of "care, cure, and coordination," which was adopted as a definition of the role of the nurse by American nurses in 1967, was given a thorough pummeling by the group. There were sharp differences among the panel members around this concept and its usefulness in defining the role of the nurse. One panel member expressed the view that if care was not the unique role of the nurse, then we all might as well give up and go home. The opposite reaction was voiced by another member: "You don't have to know anything to care . . . the janitor can care." The argument by one member that the nurse is the one whom patients can consistently count on, twenty-four hours a day, was countered by one who said that any group, for instance psychologists, if they were there twenty-four hours a day would be counted upon for that type of caring. With that statement, one of the authors pictured in her mind's eye a group of psychologists on twenty-four hour duty scurrying around taking care of patients. It was a funny picture. But why is it funny? Does it have to do with the status of women and the status of nursing, which is a little low, and if that is true, does it follow, then, that the concept of "care" falls into the same low category? At least one nursing author has contended that the concept of care connotes a feminine dependent role.[3] Twenty-four hour duty has always been a low status responsibility. It is most often the lower echelons of nursing and medicine who fall heir to the rotating shifts. Nursing is beginning to shift its emphasis, however, and perhaps the low status of *caring* will shift also. For instance, with the advent of the clinical specialist in nursing who is relatively free of administrative duties, it is not uncommon for this person, master's degree and all, to work an evening or night shift when it is necessary to increase the quality of nursing care.

---

[3] Sarosi, G. M.: A critical theory: the nurse as a fully human person, Nursing Forum 7(4):350, 1968.

As the panel members attempted to come to grips with the concept of care, cure, and coordination, it became apparent that there was no easy answer. To describe the role of the nurse in these abstract terms is very difficult. Perhaps, as Zahourek and Tower have stated, the terms care, cure, and coordination inadequately define the role of the nurse in the community mental health center.[4] These authors said that nurses do care, they do cure, and they do coordinate, but they do so in the sophisticated context of therapist, team colleague, consultant, and liaison.[5] Perhaps a fifth role should also be added, that of social change agent, as many community mental health nurses are now suggesting. Within this context of therapist, team colleague, consultant, liaison, and social change agent, the terms care, cure and coordination take on greater meaning. However, we would be remiss if we did not mention the fact that care, cure and coordination have little relevance outside the hospital setting, if this panel's discussion is any indication. In spite of the fact that nurse panelists were from community mental health centers, the terms care, cure and coordination seemed immediately to focus their attention on the inpatient setting. The panel members spent an inordinate amount of time discussing the nurse's role within this area. The fact that this focus on the nurse's role within the inpatient setting occurred may have something to do with the fact that in the past the nurse worked only in hospitals. It seems that not only is there a tendency for other disciplines to stereotype the nurse's role in terms of the hospital setting, but nurses are also having a difficult time doing otherwise. And particularly is this so when nurses try to equate their role with care, cure, and coordination. By their disagreement, the panel members seemed to be saying, "The uniform doesn't fit anymore."

A nurse is a nurse is a nurse, yes or no?

There was little agreement among the panel members regarding the educational preparation necessary for the nurse in the community mental health center. "A master's degree is the basic preparation," said one. "A diploma with experience in psychiatric nursing is quite adequate," said another. It is not surprising to note the disagreement among the panel members, for there is little agreement within nursing as a whole on this matter. The continuing dispute among nurses about diploma education versus baccalaureate education represents a great deal of ambivalence. Higher education for nurses is not valued by a significant portion of the profession. The furor created by the American Nurses' Association position paper on the educational preparation of nurses has not yet quieted down. In addition, hospital directors and

[4] Zahourek, R., and Tower, M.: Community mental health nurses question care, cure and coordination, Conference on Nursing in Community Mental Health Centers of the American Nurses' Association, 1970, American Journal of Nursing **70**(5):1021, May 1970.
[5] *Ibid*, p. 1021.

administrators have often made the statement that baccalaureate nurses are less skilled than the diploma prepared nurse. Older nurses complain about the new graduates' lack of preparation with statements such as, "They certainly didn't have to work like I did when I was in school," or "They don't have *any* clinical skill." Statements such as these demonstrate a difficulty within nursing in replacing the service model. The motto has traditionally been "learn by doing," or more to the point, "learn by doing one hundred times." Service, repetition, and self-sacrifice were the cornerstones of nursing education for many years. Nursing education has changed drastically in the last twenty years, but many of the old attitudes are still influential. In his delightful article, "The Doctor-Nurse Game," Stein describes the atmosphere of most current schools of nursing as basically restrictive.[6] While the nurses on the panel were struggling with some of these attitudes, the majority (three out of four) felt that baccalaureate preparation was the basic education for the nurse in the community mental health center. They felt that a minimum of master's degree preparation in psychiatric or mental health nursing was necessary for *optimum* development of the nurse's role in the outpatient setting. They identified a difference in emphasis between the nurse's role on the inpatient setting of a center and the outpatient setting. The panel members described their outpatient team role as primary therapists with responsibility for diagnosis and treatment of an independent caseload. The additional theoretical background of a master's degree, they felt, permitted the nurse to competently fill this role. They felt the emphasis on the inpatient setting was as co-therapist by contrast.

Another related issue regarding educational preparation was that of professional confidence. There was consensus that additional preparation at the master's level gave the nurse the theoretical armamentarium she needed to deal on a colleague basis with other members of the team. The additional background increases the nurse's confidence as well as her fund of knowledge. Nurses with less preparation can and do function on outpatient teams, but not usually, it seems, on an equal basis with other professionals in terms of shared roles and responsibilities. Whether this is a function of the nurse's self-image or the status image other professionals have of the less prepared nurse is a difficult question. Chance and Arnold provide some evidence to suggest that the differences in educational background, as well as the differences in socioeconomic background, tend to distort communication at least between doctors and nurses.[7] A conclusion by another author is that difficulties in communication "will necessarily continue until nursing makes a much needed final decision as to which type of program prepares the profes-

---

[6] Stein, L. I.: The doctor-nurse game, Archives of General Psychiatry **16**:701, June 1967.
[7] Chance, E., and Arnold, J.: The effect of professional training, experience and preference for a theoretical system upon clinical care, description, Human Relations **13**:195–213, Aug. 1960.

sional nurse."[8] This same author made another point along this line, saying, "the trend in nursing toward baccalaureate and graduate training may in time bring about considerable reduction in the educational gap between physicians and nurses. Less difficulty with the message system should be one of the end results."[9]

There are many issues raised relative to the desirable education for nurses in a community mental health center. The realities of life must be taken into consideration in terms of the number of nurses available to do the job; whether additional education humanizes, as some nurses contend, or dehumanizes, as Jourard[10] and other panel members contend; and is a nurse capable of doing the same job regardless of background. As you will recall, the panels of psychologists and psychiatrists sharply contested the question of whether additional preparation was necessary for the nurse in the outpatient setting of the community mental health center. However, there was no question in the minds of these nurses that additional preparation had made them more competent, self-confident clinicians. It does not seem that a nurse is a nurse is a nurse.

Nurses are their own worst enemies

Interestingly enough, there was disagreement on the issue of a hierarchy among professionals and nonprofessionals in the community mental health center. One nurse claimed to work in a setting in which everyone worked together as peers with equal respect paid to each person's opinion. Another nurse sharply disagreed, saying, "What system doesn't have a hierarchy? I've never worked in one that didn't." Another nurse proposed that salary defines the hierarchy. At that point the age-old gripe came into focus, namely, that nursing does not convey prestige, status, or financial reward to its practitioners. A nurse, as a general rule, cannot command equal pay with other mental health professionals even if she has equal education and experience. If nothing else, this fact proclaims the reality of the status hierarchy. In this, it seems, nurses are often their own worst enemies. In the first place, nurses block effective change in this area if they deny that the problem exists. "I don't see any top," they say while looking at their feet.

Another way in which nurses are their own worst enemies is by remaining "hung-up" eternally on the educational issue. No other profession equates technical or junior college level training with education in a university setting. How in the world, then, can nurses expect to have this stand accepted by other professionals—a nurse is a nurse is a nurse. The answer is, of course,

---

[8] Christman, *op cit*, p. 151.
[9] *Ibid*, p. 151.
[10] Jourard, S.: Speech presented at Third Annual Henrietta Loughran Seminar Series, Denver, Colorado, Jan. 27, 1970.

that nobody, including many nurses, is going to accept that stand as valid. The profession of nursing further hangs itself up with a vision of glorious ecumenicism. Nurses frequently buy the following argument from administrators: "If we change you or your level, we have to change everybody, and we can't do that now. Please wait until we can do it for everyone." The Task Force charges that this is a "cop out." The real world simply does not operate in ecumenical terms, and the hard fact is that not all members of a system can move at once. Except in rare instances, change occurs by small precedents being set. Change occurs in steps, not in leaps. Leaving an entire system bad is not better than making changes that may not affect everyone at once. It seems that a partly bad, partly good system is better than one which is all bad.

Another way that the nurses are their own worst enemy has taken form in the demand for "experience." Nurses in service agencies are unwilling to give status to education just as nurse educators are unwilling to give status to experience. As a consequence, a nurse can have a master's degree, but because she lacks "experience," she will start at a beginning staff level. No other profession, it seems, works as hard as nursing does to keep its practitioners on the bottom of the pay scale in relation to other professionals. This phenomenon has recently been described in a recent Medical World News article:

> . . .there is a strange, almost mystical ambivalence about pay. The nursing profession is perhaps the only segment of the nation's labor force that acquiesces in—and often initiates and enforces—efforts to keep down the salaries of its own members. The law of supply and demand is repeatedly ignored, and in both conversation and policy nurses repeatedly weigh their own needs against what they consider to be the needs of the society.[11]

The status of nursing consultation

The discussion of the nurse's role in consultation also brought up a status-related issue. One of the nurses recounted her experience as a consultant to a group of YMCA counselors. She said, "There is resistance to having anybody with lower status consult to someone with higher status. The group of social workers wanted a psychiatrist, but they got me instead. They seemed initially dubious and disappointed but later accepted me quite well." The other nurses on the panel also identified the difficulty nurses have had in accepting consultation from other nurses. Here again, status differences between the nurse and psychiatrist seem to play a role. However, this problem is gradually dissipating as clinical specialists become more involved in con-

---

[11] The battle over nurses, Medical World News, Nov. 21, 1969, McGraw-Hill, Inc., p. 36.

sultation.[12,13] Nurse to doctor consultation is also practiced by nurses, especially in crisis services across the country. Status issues make consultation by nurses to other professionals a touchy area. From some recent data reported at Denver General Community Mental Health Center, it seems that nurses with master's degrees feel the least prepared in this area, which adds to the problem. Nurses from other elements of the center, as reported in the study, had other concerns, but consultation was the difficult area for the outpatient team nurse.[14] Whether the problem arises from lack of knowledge or lack of status is hard to answer. The difficulty may arise as a result of both.

To summarize, it seems that nursing contributes to the problem of hierarchy and status by clinging to an antiquated set of values and by denying the presence of the issue. The issue of status relates most concretely to the issue of salary. Nurses will not get higher salaries and status until they resolve some of these issues. Certainly no other profession is going to do it for us. It is perhaps a commentary on the status of nursing that one nurse on the panel said, "It's for sure, the nurse is not regarded as an intellectual in the community." The Task Force must agree.

The chronic patient, challenge or scut work?

The connotation attached to "scut work" is that it is a disagreeable task that is given to someone low in status. Are nurses most capable of dealing with the chronic patient or is this job "scut work"? One of the nurses remarked that she gets very nervous and paranoid when she hears a doctor saying that there is "something" about a nurse that makes her the best person to care for the chronic patient. She is afraid this "something" is a willingness to do the scut work or take patients nobody else wants. In this same vein, another nurse laughed and said that whenever one staff man said he had a good patient for her, she could describe the patient before he did. Usually, she said, the patient he had in mind was a chronic schizophrenic or someone who had alienated every other professional by obnoxious behavior. Does the nurse truly have a special talent in dealing with the chronic patient, or is this an unsupported myth?

The majority of the nurses' training takes place in the hospital setting. In this setting, there are many chronically ill patients, but they are there with acute illnesses or exacerbations of chronic illness. The nurse has a great deal of experience taking care of the patient in bed, but this does not necessarily mean she gains skill in caring for the chronically ill. Public health nurses have developed skill in this area, the Task Force thinks, out of necessity. It may

---

[12] Stokes, G., and others: The roles of psychiatric nurses in community mental health practice: a giant step, New York, 1969, Faculty Press, Inc.
[13] Zahourek and Tower, *op cit.*, p. 1021.
[14] Zahourek, R.: A study of the role of nurses in a community mental health center. Unpublished study.

be that the public health nurse's expertise in this area is gained from work in the field, often after her education is completed, because those are the kinds of patients doctors and agencies refer to the public health nurse. If the referring source views the patient as a challenge and refers the patient to the nurse out of a belief in her expertise, that is one matter; if the patient, however, is referred to a nurse because she is seen as a compliant soul who will accept disagreeable tasks, that is an entirely different matter. The nurses on the panel varied in how they viewed the issue. One thought that the nurse truly does have something special to offer the chronically ill patient because the nurse is more willing to work with less tangible results and therefore tends to be more accepting. There was considerable variation of opinion among the panel members, which seemed to be due to a personal preference for a style of working. It may be true that nurses are no more knowledgeable about the care of the chronically ill patient than other professionals; however, they may be more willing to tackle the problem.

There are mental health settings in which the nurse's role concerns "aftercare." This usually means follow-up of the patient discharged from a state hospital. If a nurse prefers this kind of work, we say fine. However, if that is the only role a mental health team perceives for a nurse, it is likely that the chronic patient is viewed as scut work. If the latter is the case and the nurse who is hired does not happen to like taking care of the chronically ill any better than anyone else does, then that nurse would do well to negotiate the matter with the rest of the mental health team instead of passively accepting that definition of her role. Certainly the chronically ill patient, whether he be physically or emotionally ill, is becoming a problem of greater proportion. It is a particular problem for community mental health centers because the care of *all* patients within their own community was the mandate under which federal funds were first made available in 1963. Therefore, it seems that the chronic patient must be viewed as a challenge by all team members and not just as scut work for a nurse. In the best of all possible worlds, the care of the chronic patient will not be viewed as scut work by either the nurse or other professionals.

Handmaiden to the doctor

These nurses brought some of the status issues into focus, in part, by disagreeing about them. However, there was a unanimous discontent with the traditional role of the nurse as the handmaiden to the doctor. There was, finally, a general agreement that all settings have a hierarchy of sorts but that there is a great deal of difference in being guided by the doctor and being led around by the nose. It may be that as women gain true equality in the larger society, the idea of "handmaiden to the doctor" will just as surely disappear. This role of the nurse has developed not only because of the attitudes of doctors, primarily men, but also because of the attitudes of nurses, primarily women. The handmaiden role has met the needs of both. Dr. Stein refers to this relationship as a "transactional neurosis that is inhibitory, stifling and anti-intellectual."[15] Critics have gone on to point out that this "game" is dangerous to the patient as well.

Medical World News referred to a recent U.S. Department of Labor study that pointed to the fact that the shortage of nurses is, in part, due to the dissatisfaction of many nurses with the handmaiden role.[16] Perhaps it is time for everyone to dispense with it. Doctors will have to trade in the feeling of omnipotence the handmaiden role creates and maintains. A study comparing hospital trained nurses with baccalaureate trained nurses revealed that the hospital trained nurse had a tendency to select doctor-nurse interactions; the nurses from college schools of nursing were more likely to choose nurse-patient interactions. Perhaps it has been difficult for the physician to give up the somewhat flattering dependency of the diploma prepared nurse.[17] In return for accepting aggressiveness and independence from the nurse, the doctor will find that he has gained a competent colleague and a source of information for use in decision-making that was formerly lost in the "game." These new roles will also save time. Nurses in community mental health centers who no longer play the game of handmaiden seem to find their jobs much more rewarding and satisfying. A professional problem-solving model, such as that suggested by Miller and Sabshin in which psychiatrist-nurse-patient interaction is modeled to keep arbitrariness ("no head shall be higher than mine") at a minimum[18] warrants serious consideration in view of the problem with the current model. The relinquishment of the traditional model seems to hold the only promise for a *real* change in the role of the nurse from handmaiden to colleague.

Research—by nurses?

To the question of nurses being involved in research there was a resounding "yes" from the panel members. One panelist felt that because nursing research has often been left to other professionals, the results have had little relevance to the nurse clinician. Sharing the research role with other mental health professionals was felt to be valuable, but abdication of a role in research to other "better prepared" professionals was thoroughly discouraged by the nurses.

Regarding the educational preparation for the nurse involved in research in community mental health centers, there was good consensus. A master's

---

[15] Stein, *op cit*, p. 699.

[16] The battle over nurses, *op cit*, p. 37.

[17] Meyer, G. R.: The attitude of student nurses toward patient contact and their images of and preferences for four nursing specialties, Nursing Research 7:126–130, Oct. 1958.

[18] Miller, A. A., and others: Psychotherapy in psychiatric hospitals: a proposed model for psychiatrist-nurse-patient interaction, Archives of General Psychiatry, vol. 9, July 1963, pp. 53–63.

degree in psychiatric nursing was considered minimum basic preparation. A doctorate, the panelists felt, was ideal and a goal which needed to be set for the future. The panelist who was involved in research had a master's degree and said that she did not feel prepared to develop a lot of "highfalutin" research designs. However, she did feel prepared to do simpler kinds of clinical nursing studies and to collaborate with other professionals in the center. As a result of this nurse's research, roles of the nurse in that community mental health center have been defined much more clearly than has been possible in other centers lacking this kind of resource. The involvement of a nurse, full-time, in research in a mental health center also seemed to have stimulated many other nurses in the center to become involved in research and publication. The interest of the nurses in this center in research and publication as described by the nurse panelist was enviable. Probably the interest and activity would not have evolved had it not been for the assignment of one nurse full-time in a research-publication capacity. In this assignment she helped coordinate and encourage the efforts of the other nurses. A master's degree nurse doing full-time research? The answer seems to be a definite "yes" in terms of both capability and value to other nurses and the center as a whole.

Nurse-therapist, consultant, liaison, colleague

Another major theme around which there was solid agreement was the functional roles of the nurse in community mental health centers. The kinds of things the nurses said they did fell very well within the framework described previously by Zahourek and Tower. In this paper, as you may recall, the authors state that the concept of care, cure, and coordination has little relevance for the role of the nurse in the community mental health center. The role of the nurse, they feel, is better described as: (1) therapist, (2) consultant, (3) liaison for the patient and community agencies, and (4) team member.[19] It does seem that this description gives some clear guidelines to those who educate nurses, those who employ them, and to the individual nurse who contemplates working in a community mental health center.

Another emerging role of the nurse in the community mental health center is that of social activist or social change agent. In February 1970, nurses across the country met in New York to discuss nursing in community mental health centers. A theme in many of those discussions was the role of the nurse as a social change agent. This role was seen as being part of primary prevention. The panelists did not discuss this role; however, the Task Force will do so in the latter part of this book, because we feel that it is vitally important. Treatment and primary prevention are not mutually exclusive, and it is our

---

[19] Zahourek and Tower, *op cit.*

belief that community mental health centers can and should operate in both areas and that social change agent may well be a role for the nurse. If this statement is accurate, it has implications for nursing education as it demands a background in sociology, cultural anthropology, and social power.

At this point, the reader may well be questioning the broadness of the roles ascribed to nurses in the community mental health center. Are these legitimate roles or is the nurse, once again, trying to be all things to all people? The authors feel these are legitimate, necessary roles in the relatively new setting of the community mental health center. However, depending upon the goals of the particular center in which the nurse is employed, there may be greater emphasis on the role of therapist than there is on the role of social change agent. In describing the role of the nurse, there are few absolutes. There are many functional roles of the nurse, and they are comparable to the roles played by other professionals in the community mental health center. The panelists agreed that there should be no more handmaiden, no more bedpan stereotype, no more uniform, and no more separation as paraprofessional or ancillary personnel.

If you don't love us—fake it

As one can assume from the preceding parts of this chapter, there was unanimous agreement among the panelists that the nurse was a valuable member of the community mental health center staff. They felt she had a variety of skills comparable to those of other professionals in community mental health. In centers where nurses are currently employed in a variety of positions, the nurses are generally valued. However, convincing a new center to include nurses as part of the basic team is sometimes difficult. We know the problem well, having tried, during a panel discussion, to influence a psychiatrist to include nurses as part of the outpatient team. His feeling was that he could get a housewife to do the job a nurse could do. These nurse panelists definitely disagree with this view. If nurses are valuable and necessary members, what is it they have to offer? Read on.

The X factor

It was very interesting that after having gone through a lengthy and somewhat heated discussion about the unique role of the nurse during the first part of the interview and arriving at no consensus, the nurses came back to the same issue at the close of their discussion and reached some agreement. The question reappeared as an outgrowth of their discussion around the value of the nurse as a member of the professional staff in the community mental health center. The question hanging in the air at that point was, "Why?" The nurse shares the roles of therapist, consultant and so on, so why not hire another psychiatrist or psychologist, or social worker? The answer to that question was subtle and not easily reached. One of the panelists, after a pause said, "Well, I can't exactly identify it, but there is something holy about a patient that came to me in nurses' training. I didn't go in with 'it,' but I came out with 'it'." Another panelist called "it" the X factor. She said that she couldn't identify "it" either, but there seemed to be an X factor in the nurse's relationship to the patient. After that statement the nurses began trying to define the uniqueness of a nurse as they saw it. The medical background of the nurse was an important part of the equation. An additional factor was the eclectic nature of the nurse's educational background. The nurse specializes to some extent but is still generalist enough to see the whole patient. It was agreed that nursing education puts more emphasis on the total patient than does current medical education. One of the more elusive qualities of nurses' background is the fact that they have dealt intimately with the basics of life and death. Perhaps as a result of this, the nurse has learned to assess the realistic and practical aspects of situations. Another important factor identified by the panelists was that the nurse's basic orientation to the patient is guided also by the ethics learned as part of the profession—the "something holy." The ethics involve, ideally, a profound respect for the individual, integrity and honesty (particularly when mistakes are made), and a willingness to sacrifice one's own comfort, especially sleep, in order to provide service to the patient. These ethics are taught (or more often absorbed) during nurses' training.

Nurses, it was said, are more willing to work with less tangible results than are other professionals. The nurse, in other words, is willing to work with the patient because he needs help, not simply because she may cure him. In addition, the panelists felt nurses are definitely more practical and realistic than other professionals and, as a result, are better able to meet the patient on his own level. The unique role of the nurse is not reducible to a single word, such as care, but *educated caring* comes as close as any term in describing the uniqueness of her role. In all, the X factor seems to be composed of regard for the patient, a practical orientation, and the ability to be satisfied with helping.

Summary

Were these nurses out of uniform and into trouble? If trouble is controversy, discontent with the traditional role of the nurse, expansion into new roles, greater professional independence and satisfaction, then the answer is yes, and it's a good kind of trouble.

The interesting aspects of this discussion were the controversy about the concept of care and about the educational preparation of nurses, the rejection of the traditional role of handmaiden to the doctor, the confidence they felt in their ability to fulfill new roles, and the X factor or uniqueness of a nurse. We think they demonstrated quite well why nurses should be members of the community mental health team and why the big three may need to give way to the big four. Nurses are capable professionals who are no longer content with traditional roles only or second-class status. The nurse has a special background that is valuable to a community mental health team and, more importantly, to the patient.

Chapter Nine

NURSE ADMINISTRATORS— THE CHIEFS' POW-WOW

Two administrators, one from a large mental health center and the other representing a health department, met simultaneously with the nurse educators, although for purposes of presentation they will be discussed separately. Of all the groups interviewed, these interviewees were the most constrained. As authors, we postulated this restrained discussion might be due to two things. One, administrators deal daily with ponderous problems without a lot of "horse-play." Consequently, in the interview they dealt with issues in the same straightforward, humorless manner. Second, the traditional animosity between service and education seemed to be in evidence with this combined group. The animosity could explain the lack of humor. Perhaps we, as investigators, had desired to witness a fight, but in retrospect we feel it was a poor choice of groupings.

In order to gain further information about administrators' views, a nursing director of a community mental health center, an associate director of a health department, and a nursing director of a teaching psychiatric hospital were queried at a later date.

Nursing is in an oblong box

"We're boxed in," a director commented. Some of this box's lumber is really made up by the profession itself. This director pointed out that one of the factors boxing nursing in is the Nurse Practice Acts, which in most states are twenty-five years outdated. These outdated Acts unfortunately restrict the nursing services, especially in the field of psychiatry.

Stachyra studied the national problem of Nurse Practice Acts, and pointed out that in many states nurses are inhibited in their individual practice of psychotherapy. She identified the problem as being twofold. First, that the definition of psychotherapy is loose in most states; none of the fifty states' nursing laws clearly states that psychotherapy is a part of the "professional nursing" definition. Second, that practicing as a nurse under the supervision of a physician restricts independent functioning. Stachyra concludes that in many instances the nurse has more freedom practicing as a "psychotherapist" rather than as a "nurse." She also identifies an additional problem, that of the same licensure for all levels of academic preparation.[1] In her conclusion, Stachyra delineates three specific areas of practice acts which should receive

---

[1] Stachyra, M.: Nurses, psychotherapy, and the law, Perspectives in Psychiatric Care **8**:200–213, 1969.

remedial action. They are "(1) provision for practice at different levels of nursing—the nurse with a master's or doctorate degree being qualified to perform beyond the limits of nurses with less preparation; (2) specific naming of the independent practice of psychotherapy as a function of educationally qualified nurses; (3) specific mention of the supervision of the physician over nurses. Finally, repeal any act which is unduly restrictive of a nursing function would not be too rash a goal."[2]

Another director viewed the Nurse Practice Acts as further curtailing the nurse's functioning by encumbering her with supervisory responsibilities of subprofessionals such as psychiatric technicians. This director confessed that staffing a large state hospital with twenty-four hour coverage by registered nurses on each unit was not feasible. The need for rotating shifts and weekend coverage stripped the staff to a bare minimum. In essence, the law was being broken, and both the state hospital and the State Board of Nurse Examiners knew the "unlawful" situation existed but they were making the best of a bad situation.

In contrast, an administrator pointed to the flexibility of the Mental Health Worker's role. This worker, who has an associate arts degree, is not curtailed by legislation either to be directly under the supervision of the physician or is he responsible for the acts of subprofessionals. She pointed out that the freedom of the nurse to move in and out of the hospital setting is hampered. "How can they [nurses] do intakes in the community or participate in community liaison work with a narcotics key around their necks?" Readers may, as did the authors, see this as a cop-out. Why not give the keys to the directors of nursing and really be flexible!

Streamlining services

The administrators felt the duplication of services should be eliminated. For instance, they noted that home visits were being done by both the mental health center and the health department. Less dichotomizing of all service was advocated. Another director yearned for a revolution of the total health care system. As she said, "Right now we have a *no care* system." She advocated new studies in sociology and anthropology to stimulate broader thinking about tired, old problems. "We're in a rut and need new inputs into nursing," she concluded.

A need to change our total health care system has many supporters. One of the most articulate is Peter Rogatz who characterizes the existing health programs as a "non-system." One of the fundamental detriments to our present policies, he feels, is the unilateral decisions which are made regarding health care. These decisions are made without the participation or represen-

---

[2] *Ibid*, p. 213.

tation of the consumer. He calls for a change in the "closed" system in which roles are stereotyped and rigid to a new system in which the public consumer involvement is fully implemented and utilized.[3]

Public health nursing and psychiatric nursing— a place for both?

In attempting to differentiate between the functions of public health nurses and psychiatric nurses, one director viewed a combined role and labeled this nurse a "community mental health nurse." She believed that kinds of therapies such as group, individual, milieu, and home visits utilized nursing skills, but that the orientation toward meeting *total* health needs was the community mental health nurse's role. Using this connotation of the word role, there would be no duplication of public healh nurses' and psychiatric nurses' services. The core nursing role was defined as "the ability to aid the patient in new perceptions of self and insight into changed patterns of behavior." The nurse has the opportunity, because of continuous contact with the patient, to provide repetitive kinds of learning that comes with practicing new behaviors and ways of relating to others. She has opportunities for supervising experiences in living—not only in an institutional setting but also in the community. She should be able to move back and forth between settings without the barriers of walls. However, moving back and forth between hospital and community settings is more ideal than real. As was alluded to before, one administrator argued that shortage of staff prevented psychiatric nurses from going into the community. Another director countered that this argument was a rationalization. Her hypothesis was that the traditional inpatient psychiatric nurse does not venture into the community because (1) it is frightening to leave the familiar structure of the hospital; (2) it carries little reward from the inpatient psychiatric team.

Another saw that psychiatric nurses really did not trust the public health nurses. She said, "Many psychiatric nurses will say public health nurses don't know beans about psychiatry but that these public health nurses really have the inroads to the family." Others gave the public health nurses credit for their special abilities to assess family situations. Not all agreed with this, however, and it was argued (with no conclusion) that the public health nurses were really afraid of family dynamics and so were psychiatric nurses. It was felt nurses generally lacked knowledge about family crisis intervention. The big question was: where should this knowledge be gained? Most of these nurses lacked master's degrees, so it was suggested that continuing education programs with special supervision be tried.

Another important issue was raised. It was noted that public health nurses

---

[3] Rogatz, P.: The health care system, Hospitals **44:**47–50, 1970.

and psychiatric nurses viewed each other's arenas as "the grass is greener on the other side." For instance, the public health nurse expressed ambivalence at being an independent practitioner. On the one hand she liked her "freedom," but on the other hand, she was afraid of it: "I'm all alone here, frustrated, and feeling inadequate with this patient." The public health nurse was also expected to seek out other resources, which in some agencies were nonexistent.

In contrast, the psychiatric nurse envied the free agent status of the public health nurse. The inpatient setting was viewed as a closed system in which roles and alliances were rigidly fixed. "Learning the system takes all her time and energy," was one comment. Another opinion was that the nurse working in the inpatient setting had so many alliances and reference groups that the patient got left out. An incident, which is not rare, happened on a hospital unit when a team was attempting to solve some team interpersonal problems. They were expending so much energy in this endeavor that the patients were neglected. This neglect was viewed by one patient as rejection or an invitation to death, and he committed suicide. This phenomenon is discussed by Sidney Jourard in his article, "Invitation to Die."[4]

Staffing the setting

Concerning staffing their departments or hospitals, the administrators believed that the philosophies of each agency attracted different graduates with different goals for their nursing careers. In hiring new staff, one administrator relied heavily upon the personality traits of the individual. She was concerned about the ability of the new staff nurse to be innovative and her commitment to nursing. This administrator held little confidence in grades earned in nursing education, since "They only reflect the grading system of that one school and are not comparable with other schools."

"Hiring a large number of bright enthusiastic new graduates may seem to be ideal, but I have found too many new graduates are a drain on the staff," commented a director. She pointed out that the amount of time and effort expended in orienting new staff was tremendous and that new graduates hadn't yet "settled down" before they moved on to other positions. Staff turnover is an eternal problem. This director balanced her staff with new graduates and old-timers. She also noted that hiring associate degree graduates posed problems. Although many of them have more clinical hours in their psychiatric preparation, they were graduated at a young age, and this director found them immature. She also noted the need to provide an "internship" for them, which was a costly budgeting problem.

Another administrator had encountered the problem of hiring nurses with

---

[4] Jourard, S. M.: Suicide—the invitation to die, American Journal of Nursing **70**(2):269–275, Feb. 1970.

advanced preparation. This change had riled the sytem on all sides. First, she had to bang heads with hospital administrators and the civil service bureaucracy in order to establish a justifiable salary for the educational level. Then she needed to fight the brush fires of the staff nurses who were threatened on several counts such as (1) do I have to go back to school to keep my job; (2) what does this nurse know that I don't; and (3) is the system going to test me as to my skills? Fighting the issues on both sides is one of the biggest challenges of the nursing administrator's position.

Recruiting in this metropolitan area created no problems for the administrators at that time. Those in the rural areas were not so fortunate. In this metropolitan area an abundance of highly specialized clinicians were applying for openings in a new, creative Model Cities program. There has been a national shift in the occupation of the fifteen hundred nurses who have been prepared in master's programs.[5] One half are teaching and the other half are in clinical work settings. Service agencies used to have a difficult time competing with educational settings for master's prepared nurses. The pay scale was lower and working conditions less desirable. However, in the Denver area, the trend is reversing as new clinical specialists are seeking the creative jobs in community psychiatry.

A comment on nursing education

Although none of the administrators was directly involved with classroom teaching, each was very involved with providing clinical experiences for both basic undergraduate and graduate nurse education. Furthermore, their agencies and institutions were utilized by a variety of students in the mental health field. They were concerned about the quality of education and also the end product—the staff they hire.

The question of the most desirable academic preparation for community mental health center nurses created a controversy. One administrator was convinced that the minimum preparation for a nurse to function in an outpatient setting was a master's degree, for in this setting the complexity of problems demanded a nurse with greater special preparation. Others questioned the use of such a nurse for direct patient care rather than for consultation. Educational preparation was not important to another who viewed individual skills, personality, and interest as the most important attributes in hiring staff.

How to kill creativity

The chance of a nurse retaining her creativity after exposure to basic nursing education was viewed dimly. As one stated, "Nursing education kills crea-

---

[5] Stachyra, *op cit*, p. 201.

tivity." Another continued, "We need a greater depth of understanding of clinical psychiatry. Many schools focus on interpersonal relationships and communication skills, but not enough focus on clinical nursing." For instance, being able to manage a total unit of withdrawn, acting out, or aggressive patients demands more skill in assessment, making clinical judgments, and collaborating with a team than the simplistic understanding of initiating and terminating a relationship. Nursing education, she said, needs to focus more on broader concepts of organization. They need to change their attitudes about working with other disciplines. "They need to develop the attitude of working as a peer and not as a subordinate."

Another expressed more concern about the role models the student has. She said, "There are no real models for the nursing student, as the staff nurse is too enmeshed in the organization's hierarchy and the instructor is too rigid in wanting it done her way." There is a pitiful lack of communication between the staff nurse and the instructor. The student, however, catches the flack in the middle. Attempts toward opening communication between the staff nurse and the instructor is the heart of the problem. In the diploma schools there were advantages in having the director of the school and the director of the nursing service as one person. The lines of communication were very direct, and the staff nurse had a definite function in role modeling regardless of whether or not the model was a good one.

The rigidity of nursing education came up as a continual thread of concern. Could it be that working with and molding the new graduate into a productive staff member gives rise to this choleric attitude? Had administrators really experienced such bad products, or were they Monday morning quarterbacking? One summarized by saying, "Nursing education kills a lot of spontaneity and programs in a lot of assumptions that never get tested. The new staff nurse too often goes into a setting with preconceived ideas of what is operational for that system." No doubt, part of this learning is a matter of maturation on which no school has a head start. Even the more seasoned nurse has adjustments to make in assuming a new staff position. A period of readjustment to the role should be expected for all new personnel. Another result of rigidity in nursing education that is noticeable not just in the new graduate but in many experienced nurses is the fear of authority; supervision is perceived as a threat rather than a growth-producing experience.

Teaching too little in four years

Administrators were disturbed that four-year nursing students and those with master's preparation were not functioning at a higher level. As one stated, "In seven months you can train psychiatric technicians to perform at levels which exceed the graduate with a bachelor's degree." One should question what was meant by train and perform, for without a doubt it does remind one of a circus dog. In defense of baccalaureate programs, it should be pointed out that in most schools the amount of actual special education in psychiatric nursing is eight to twelve weeks! Some master's programs are only two months longer than the training program for psychiatric technicians—or nine months in all. Perhaps it is unwise to attempt to compare length of time with exit performances without identifying depth and breadth of knowledge of the graduates. It is similar to comparing apples and oranges.

During this discussion one had the sensation of attending the Mad Tea Party in Carroll's *Alice in Wonderland*. In the opening paragraph of that chapter, the March Hare and the Hatter are at the tea table with the Dormouse fast asleep between them. The March Hare and the Hatter are "resting their elbows on the Dormouse, and talking over its head." Alice thought how very uncomfortable it was for the Dormouse. It is not difficult for us to see the March Hare and Hatter as nursing service and nursing education, with the practitioner of nursing as the Dormouse. In attempting to lessen the gap between service and education, it might be well to involve the Dormouse.

Summary

In this panel discussion, little seemed to be accomplished other than giving an opening to nursing administrators to vent their spleen on nursing educators. Little in the way of real dialogue or repartee occurred which, sadly, is the rule rather than the exception. The dicussion on the value of utilizing a nurse skilled in mental health and public health in both the mental health center and the public health setting to bridge some of the misconceptions in both settings for better comprehensive patient care was also alluded to.

Chapter Ten

NURSE EDUCATORS— THE IVORY TOWER SYNDROME

The ivory tower syndrome has been a diagnostic label placed on educators. In this study it refers particularly to nursing educators. Educators have been accused of teaching because they are not capable of "doing." Being capable of expert clinical practice is highly prized talent by both students and staff nurses. If the educator does not have clinical practice or close ties with the clinical agencies, he is accused of teaching outdated and irrelevant practices. The three educators we interviewed were not outdated and irrelevant. They represented diploma, baccalaureate, and graduate programs and were articulate, animated, and argumentative. The most violent arguments surrounded the topics of nursing research and supervision of students. In addition to interviewing these educators, anecdotes were collected by the Task Force from various nurse educators and students during this period of study.

Relevant or retarded

Today our total educational system is being challenged. Questions are being raised about the relevancy of all education. Some challenges seem to arise from a naive wish to return to the simplistic one-room schoolhouse. Other challenges arise from choleric people who rebel for the sake of rebelling. Still other challenges come from an aroused populace who recognizes the need for replacing outdated practices with innovative *thinking* in the belief that if a system is sound, it has the capability of responding to change. These same challenges were verbalized by the educators interviewed. How relevant is nursing education? "We're twenty-five years or so behind the needs of society," said one educator. Being behind was blamed on (1) passive students, (2) passive nursing culture, and (3) an inflexible health care system.

Others had blamed nursing education for being too rigid, too punitive, and too irrelevant. One could conclude from many statements that it would have been better for the student nurse never to have entered the educational program. However, one educator viewed the problem as needing changes from all sides. She stated, "We are held in by a culture of nursing which resists change. I see little hope with today's students, as there are no risk takers. I'm sick to death of passive students."

However, another blamed nursing for fostering group consensus. Does any other profession always need *group consensus* before action is taken? Group consensus can operate by whittling away at individuality. Diversity is replaced with a watered down mediocre group opinion. Group consensus is evidenced at all levels of nursing, not only in educational settings. Is this quality innate in the prenursing student, or does it develop during the educational process? Corwin and Taves studied this question and found that the ideologies of prenursing students were similar to those of students in general. They noted that studies in the past had indicated that nursing attracted highly committed, dedicated students who were extremely idealistic in their humanitarian goals. In contrast, today's recruits for nursing are more similar to other entering college students in regard to their idealism and humanitarianism. In fact, they are more and more like students who choose other academic fields of study.[1]

This fact may mean hope for nursing. At least it indicates some change. Therefore, according to the Corwin and Taves study, this socialization process occurs *during* the nursing education and is not an innate quality. According to one student questioned by one of the authors, group consensus begins with the fear that is instilled—fear that independent action or action contrary to that sanctioned by the faculty will reap punitive results. Punitive results may be very subtle, such as, low grades or the connotation of being a "bad" student, and therefore a "bad" nurse. So well socialized are some students in this passive role that one claimed, "Things are black or white depending on what the instructor says." Another graduating senior retorted, "After two years I didn't know I was capable of having an opinion of my own!"

The group consensus phenomenon pervades other areas of nursing besides the student population. As one nurse educator claimed, "The trouble with us [nurses] is that we've gotten ourselves into a thimble." A thimble has a way out, but it's put on by the wearer for self-protection. Perhaps this self-protection has made us pretty dull, and a few pin pricks may help to change our rigid mold. Or, "Are we going to be comfortable with marginality?" asked another educator. Being on the margin is a safe place, but dull if you want the center column. Margins do serve to define parameters for the main body of a story, but margins are pretty narrow and drab; besides, other people may doodle in them! So, let some fur fly—open arenas can be much more fun than a telephone booth. "Flexibility in the nursing culture should be perpetuated on all sides—even students as well as deans may be spinning their wheels in well-worn ruts," commented a professor.

The broad-bottomed nurse

Throughout this study interviewees have either praised the fact that nursing education is based upon a broad field of knowledge and practice, or they have been alarmed that because it is so broadly based, there is no clearly, well-defined body of knowledge and skill. These interviewees agreed that the broad-base knowledge of nursing education was an asset for practice. Because

---

[1] Corwin, R. G., and Taves, M. J.: Nursing and other health professions. In Freeman, H. E., Levine, S., and Reeder, L. G., editors: Handbook of medical sociology, Englewood Cliffs, N.J., 1963, Prentice-Hall, Inc., pp. 187–212.

of this knowledge, the nurse should be better prepared to translate total needs of the patient, especially for nonmedical members of the team. An incident supporting this belief was cited by one educator. She had been asked by a social worker to consult with a depressed young mother who was overly anxious about caring for the colostomy of her three-year-old daughter. This social worker was competent in family therapy, but she recognized much of the mother's anxiety and depression centered around the lack of skill and confidence in performing this nursing task.

Nursing does have a holistic approach to man. This aspect of functioning has been discussed in several of the preceding chapters. Being able to help the patient "keep body and soul together" was the way one educator described this broadly based educational process.

Another important aspect of a broadly based education pertained to the managerial skills of a graduate nurse. The educators recognized this was one of their goals, but they questioned if today's beginning practitioner is being prepared for this function. One claimed, "The registered nurse needs ability to create a therapeutic milieu twenty-four hours a day, seven days a week. A lot of this skill is also dealing with nonpatients." Another retorted, "We talk a lot about the need for this, but we don't do a thing about teaching it." This stimulated a noted educator to point out her personal philosophy of teaching students to relate well with one patient and to understand the ramifications of object relations. She claimed if the student was clear in her understanding of the usefulness of this one-to-one skill she would be able to translate this knowledge more broadly. The practitioner could transfer the principles of a one-to-one relationship to team and total milieu management. This educator favored strongly an internship for newly graduated baccalaureate nurses under the supervision of a "master" nurse in order to gain further skill. ("Master" nurse implied a skilled nurse, and did not limit the description to a level of academic preparation.)

The cries of the student nurses are getting louder about the lack of practical experience they are getting. They even had the guts to voice the issue at the American Nurses' Association biennial convention in Miami, 1970. Perhaps if they keep crying long enough and loud enough even the "theoretical" ears of the educators will begin to listen. The diploma graduate had plenty of opportunity to gain practice when she had evening, night, and weekend clinical assignments. Her assignments were not on the aide or practical nurse level; she had responsibility of large units, which forced her to utilize managerial skills. Perhaps baccalaureate graduates, too, would gain profitable knowledge by being team leaders more often on evening, night, and weekend shifts.

Continuing in the discussion of the broad base of undergraduate education, one interviewee discussed the level of functioning nurses had in group settings. Several others agreed that nurses possessed superior group skills. The educators were recognizing the comfort level nurses have with informal groups.

This level of comfort has developed as a result of the number of group encounters the nurse experiences from the beginning of her nursing education. These informal groups are found in the hospital, such as on wards, and in diabetes and baby care classes. Clinic settings of various kinds offer group experiences. Home visits, a part of community health, also offer opportunities for group encounters.

Prevention of illness is a part of all nursing curricula, and all agreed that nurses should be skilled in preventive medicine. We also believe nurses *should* be skilled but, alas, how little skill is *really* being used in preventing illness, especially mental illness?

Closeness or intimacy was also discussed as a part of nursing education. Experientially, nurses have shared intimate moments with the people known as patients. These intimate moments are as varied as the birth of a perfect baby, the death of a loving husband, the removal of a tumor—lab report negative, or the decision to therapeutically abort an unwanted pregnancy. The educators' opinion varied as to how these experiences affected the nurse. There were several opinions expressed as to what was meant by intimacy. It was agreed that the rendering of intimate services, such as bed baths and enemas, did not necessarily make a nurse "close" to a patient. There was more agreement that sharing certain life experiences made for closeness and that not all nurses were sensitive, but that the potential for sharing and being close was there.

"If you really cared"

Are nurses caring people? As a subgroup, these educators did not comment much on this subject, and it was noted by the authors that few instructors verbalize their "caring" about patients. They did comment about their "caring" for or disliking students, but seldom patients! Perhaps students are their life's work, their reference point. However, it was a phenomenon noted with this group. Could these educators be more interested in the "head stuff" rather than the "heart stuff"? Or perhaps they are more realistic. As one said, "The desire to help people isn't all you need. Some people have said that nurses are more apt than other professions to share of *themselves*. This is an overgeneralization, as some nurses are the most hostile, cold, diluted people of all."

In this same vein, it was noted that the nurse seemed better qualified to help patients adapt to illness than to wellness. Is this observation justified? Perhaps this quality, too, may have been gained through prolonged contact with the patient in hospital settings in contrast to the relatively brief contact other disciplines have with patients. However, it is questionable if this special skill of nurses will continue as the nursing contacts are becoming noticeably briefer with the advent of treatment modalities such as crisis intervention and partial hospitalization.

It has been postulated by some writers that the "caring" nurse may actually be detrimental to the patients if caring is used in the context of mother-surrogate. If in the traditional mother-surrogate role, the nurse "cares" for the patient not as a person but as a child, this nurse meets her own egotistical needs. Instead, the really caring nurse fosters independence of the human being who is in the patient role.[2]

Generalist versus specialist issues

In discussing the issue of levels of functioning appropriate to the different types of nursing preparation, there was greater consensus with this group of interviewees. Perhaps it is more easily differentiated on paper and in course objectives than in a real-life clinical situation. Be that as it may, these educators agreed that on an undergraduate level, a specialized generalist was being prepared. This term conveyed the belief that the four-year graduate was able to function broadly in all areas of nursing, including psychiatry. Her special role, then, was as a generalist.

The basic baccalaureate nursing program includes theory and practice in community or public health nursing. Several other disciplines throughout this study had commented about the ease and comfort nurses seemingly have in making home visits. Nurse educators agreed with this observation and pointed out that this skill may have been gained from the public health experience in nursing education. Another educator felt that because the nurse was accustomed to sharing daily living experiences with patients in the hospital, the transition from the hospital to the home presented fewer barriers to her than to members of other disciplines. One stated, "Nurses know more about daily living experiences and their relationship to the total disease process, and they utilize these knowledges in caring for mental patients." Another commented, "We've been making home visits since the beginning of nursing; in fact, that's where it all began—now it's become a neat thing to do." However, one disagreed that home visits had become "a neat thing," as she had observed home visits are really low priority, low status functions in the setting where she teaches. She reasoned that, "There is little concern about how the visit went and no call for feedback from the team. It's not a high visibility function and, therefore, receives very few staff rewards." Maybe this is a reason why other disciplines perpetuate the myth of the "great" public health nurse home visitors—they don't want to do them themselves.

Graduate education was seen as a specialized education in one clinical specialty. The clinical specialist in psychiatric nursing was being prepared as an individual therapist, group therapist, and family therapist. Special skills in teaching, consultation, and administration were electives that each graduate student could choose in order to have greater depth of study.

---

[2] Sarosi, G. M.: A critical theory; the nurse as a fully human person, Nursing Forum **7**:349–362, 1960.

No attempt was made in this dialogue to differentiate exit performances of diploma graduates versus those of associate degree or baccalaureate graduates. To date, no national nursing group has been able to differentiate this difference. Several independent nurse researchers have compiled graduation charts showing levels of functioning according to preparation. One study by Messick and Aguilera utilizes four levels: R.N.; R.N., B.S; R.N., M.S; R.N., Ph.D.[3] Another paper by Gebbie, Delougherty, and Neuman discusses the levels of preparation for nurses who are prepared in community organization and consultation. They saw the framework they proposed as being useful in planning for the role of nurses in community mental health. These writers utilized a framework in which the R.N., Ph.D. was recognized as a community specialist, whose goal was comprehensive and preventive planning. This specialist focused her action in the community power structure. The next specialist was the R.N.,M.S. who was primarily a nurse clinician. This specialist concentrated her efforts on members of the community and nonmental health professionals. The third specialist, R.N.,B.S., was a specialist in psychiatric nursing. Her area of contact was with the nurse generalists.[4] These delineations of levels are useful, and certainly need much more application and reality testing.

Squelched brain syndrome—or nursing research

"Graduate students, faculty, and clinicians are gun-shy when it comes to doing research," claimed a nursing researcher. One reason given is the stereotype of nursing research. It is negative! Zero! "Not only is it rough to do," claimed another, "but other disciplines degrade nursing research as being 'too loose'. But I'm dealing with nursing situations and am not at all concerned about what *other* disciplines conclude." She emphasized the fact that clinical research using human subjects should reflect a certain 'looseness'. Nurses have untapped clinical data upon which to conduct research. It seems they lack the skill of drawing this body of data into concepts translatable to others. Confidence is also lacking that the findings will stand up under scientific scrutiny. One researcher lamented the fact that too many viewed clinical research as problem solving. Finding an answer to a problem was seen as the essence of research when, in fact, it should be drawing together facts about an observed phenomenon.

Another faculty member dimly viewed the amount of research being done. She saw that most of it was done in graduate education, and she felt innovative, inquisitive thinking was squelched. As she stated, "Graduate school is the

---

[3] Messick J., and Aguilera, D.: Realistic utilization; levels of preparation, Journal of Psychiatric Nursing, May–June 1968, pp. 133–137.
[4] Gebbie, K. M., Delougherty, G., and Neuman, B. M.: Levels of utilization: nursing specialists in community mental health, Journal of Psychiatric Nursing 8(1):37–39, Jan.–Feb. 1970.

most damaging in its rigidity and conformity." However, another member strongly argued that master's theses by and large do not bring about new knowledge but that the real learning that goes on is the disciplined approach to gathering research information. An exciting proposal was made that graduate students assist a scholarly, skilled nurse researcher (and they do exist, contrary to false rumors). Studying under the mentorship of such scholars may not be as profitable monetarily as the present grants and fellowship programs, but it could be so designed. Other professions have made great advances with this apprentice approach to research.

Another noted breakthrough in nursing research is the amount and quality of clinical research coming from the clinical specialists. They are "where the action is" and clinicians are becoming much more assertive in their publishing efforts. The best part is they are researching and *publishing* because they love it and feel they have some messages. Take note of the number of clinicians speaking out through this book! There is no threat of "publish or perish" hanging over their heads!

There's a reason why we're splitting a gut

The nursing educators were polarized. Does nursing education teach *functional* areas of practice or, instead, is the educative *process* the prime modus operandi? This argument continues on the national scene as well. The functionalists argued that obtaining knowledge and skills was the chief goal of nursing education. With the concise, well-defined body of knowledge, a practitioner, undergraduate or graduate, gained the *confidence* of a practitioner at various levels. The process supporters claimed all education was a process and that nursing education prepared a practitioner to *think* in a problem-solving and, hopefully, creative manner. These battlers claimed functional roles were limiting and the process approach was dynamic and creative. Neither side won—both are still arguing.

Both sides recognized the importance of utilizing clinical role models in their teaching. The instructor-student relationship was only a small part compared to the gestalt of the health care system.

The educators also recognized the tremendous tension within a health care system. Many other disciplines have alluded to this state of tension. L. M. Smith sheds some light on the rationale for this situation. He notes that the nurse deals with the *total* individual, which includes cultural, psychological, sociological, and biological components. The nurse must be both a humanist and natural scientist. The humanist endorses the belief that each man is a unique entity in this universe. The natural scientist finds that man is reducible to a set of natural laws, and, if he is studied closely enough, is indistinguishable from the universe. The psychiatric nurse is in the center of this continuum. On the one hand, she believes in the uniqueness of individual man, and on the other, she practices the science of nursing according to a vast array of scientific theories! Being in the middle, the nurse pulls on both sides and is in an uncomfortable tension spot.[5] Have you checked your incision lately? We recommend all nurses consult their horoscopes, and if they are not Libras, who constantly strive to maintain balance, forget it.

Overdependency—a reality or myth?

What a row this produced! The real issue was how much independence a student should have in a clinical setting. One instructor believed that students should be supervised less and allowed more freedom—even to make mistakes. Another countered, this was a dangerous attitude as it could be harmful to the patient if mistakes were made on him! He stated, "You can misuse patients even if your intentions are good. As an instructor I wouldn't turn students loose without close supervision because I have responsibilities to the patient." Perhaps some modification of *how* the supervision was carried out was the crux of the problem, as all the educators agreed students needed guidance, direction, and inspiration, not surveillance.

Is psychiatric nursing really a part of nursing?

Although this question is avoided often, it remains the crux of many problems in nursing education today. Many nursing educators do not see psychiatric nursing as a part of nursing at all. They cannot identify much in the psychiatric nurse's role that is basic to nursing. This philosophy pervades many schools throughout the country. It seems a downright peculiar attitude when over fifty percent of the hospital beds in the United States are occupied by mental patients. Maybe if mental illness is ignored, it will just go away! This attitude within schools of nursing curtails the skills of the educator. Teaching psychiatric nursing presents problems in teaching and role modeling not found in other clinical specialities such as medical, surgical, or obstetrics, where many technical skills can be demonstrated and learned. In psychiatric nursing, the very essence of the problem makes approaching the patient difficult. Having poor interpersonal relationships is a prime symptom of mental patients. Developing a therapeutic relationship takes time, much collaborating with team members, and a great deal of support and supervision from faculty. Faculty ratios cannot be the same as utilized in other clinical areas. Furthermore, lecture content includes not only facts for the cognitive domain (theories about schizophrenia) but also facts for the affective domain (how do you feel intervening with an aggressive patient?). In psychiatric nursing the instructor finds she deals more in the humanism portion of the continuum, not only with a unique, individual patient but also with a unique, individual student.

---

[5] Smith, L. M.: The system—barriers to quality nursing. In Folta, J. R., and Deck, E. S., editors: A sociological framework for patient care, New York, 1966, John Wiley & Sons, Inc., pp. 134–144.

Faculty commented upon the education toward a "generalist" goal as presenting some problems, as all students were required to take psychiatry although they were not interested. In fact, some students hated psychiatry with a passion. Creating positive learning taxed the ingenuity of the educators.

Another dilemma is being faced. It has been proposed in some schools of nursing that no special psychiatric experience is needed. It is reasoned that the object relation skills needed in psychiatry could be learned as effectively in a general hospital setting. "People are people anywhere" is the rationale. One educator asked in rebuttal, "Could a nursing student have her total cardiology experience on a psychiatric ward?" Although the educators agreed that it was necessary to learn about behavior of patients in all areas of nursing, they felt that a special psychiatric nursing experience was justifiable because it enabled the students to deal interpersonally with patients in a different way than that practiced on a general unit.

The future of psychiatry is unpredictable. Will we continue to see psychiatric patients in inpatient settings at all? Some nursing and mental health leaders have predicted that within five years there will be no large inpatient settings and that psychiatric nursing will be practiced almost totally in the community. The days of a specialized psychiatric experience may be limited in the future to a field visit to some setting where a few regressed patients are living. How true this statement is remains to be seen. It is apparent that nursing should understand more about social systems. As one educator said, "We should be teaching students much more on systems analysis." As nursing has responded toward an expanded role, the nurse has discovered she is very naive about power struggles and politics. As one educator said, "We need to identify the power in a system and to utilize this power in creating the role which is needed." Perhaps nursing curricula should include some solid courses in politics such as "War," "Machiavellian Strategies," and "Coping and Cunning."

Speed kills

Too often in these interviews were heard such comments as, "We need to catch up, or we'll be left out." Stop! We *are* making progress, but let's begin to put our best brains to use for the greatest return. The greatest return may be found at the gut level reorganization of the nursing educational hierarchy. Why not put Ph.D, full professors, charismatic educators designing and teaching nursing fundamentals where the student first encounters nursing. Let's reverse the trend of a one-to-one professor to graduate student ratio and make the professor-to-student ratio much lower on the undergraduate level instead. The cookie cutter approach, as we too often have witnessed in nursing education; such as, Nurse A^1 is like Nurse A^2, like Nurse A^3, etc., etc., etc., must yield to flexibility and creativity. Entrance requirements should be modified drastically. Let's, with due haste and courage, not lose environmentally deprived creative students because of rigid, unrealistic entrance requirements. Exit standards may remain the same, but why not take a fresh look at them, too? How do these standards help the contemporary student practice nursing in today's society and prepare her to be flexible and creative in meeting tomorrow's needs?

PART FOUR
The panorama

Chapter Eleven

MIRROR, MIRROR ON THE WALL

The reflection as we see ourselves and are seen by others, at times, has seemed to come from a mirror or a deep pool being at times crystal clear, sometimes ruffled and murky. Perhaps we (the Task Force) have been akin to the vain stepsister, saying, "Mirror, mirror on the wall, who's the fairest of them all," and wanting to hear the other disciplines say, "you." That nurses were the fairest of them all is not what we heard, nor is it probably what we needed to hear. What the mirror reflected has been both positive and negative and, therefore, of benefit to the Task Force in our attempt to understand the role of the nurse in the community mental health center. Many factors affect this role, as was postulated in the beginning. In these concluding chapters, we will comment on the themes that seemed most relevant.

The pecking order

The ways in which we are seen by all levels of mental health workers affect our role performance. As a professional group, it becomes essential that we understand what other groups think about us. This does not, or should it, mean that people other than ourselves define what our education should be or what our role, based on that body of education, should be. It merely means that the recognition of how others see us affects our role expectations as well as our performance and places us in a better position to learn, not only how to cope with our position in the pecking order, but possibly how to effect changes in that ranking and allow others to do the same.

The rank and file of the mental health team lines up in a certain order from "high" man to "low" man. The ranking usually places the psychiatrist at the top with the psychologist, social worker, nurse, and technician or aide lining up in that order. In a general hospital setting, the ranking would be similar, although the disciplinary names might differ. Holding up the rear, even if you were to add such disciplines as nutritionist, vocational rehabilitation, and occupational therapists to the team, you would still find the nurse and the technician. This team ranking is called by many the "pecking order." Pecking order, as defined by Webster's dictionary, refers to "the basic pattern of sound organization within a flock of poultry in which each kind pecks another lower in the scale without fear of retaliation and submits to pecking by one of higher rank." This kind of social organization is not unusual. It is found with rare exceptions in most organizations and businesses as well as in chicken coops. It is also found in most of the community mental health center teams to which we have been exposed.

What is unusual about the community mental health center teams and the nurses on those teams is the frequent denial of the reality of the hierarchical ranking or pecking order. It is frequently said, and occasionally, but rarely true, that everyone on a team has an equal say in patient treatment, or anyone on the teams in the mental health center can become the team leader, even a nurse or technician.

Is there a realistic in-between? This is difficult to answer. You have seen in the preceding chapters that the varying ways people view the nurse influences her place on the team. Sometimes she "pecks." More often she is "pecked" upon. On occasion, she is not even on the team. Is this issue important? Can it possibly make any difference to the delivery of mental health services as to whether or not nurses are involved in that delivery? Furthermore, even if it makes a difference, does it matter in which way they are involved so long as they are involved at some level? We think it does matter on both counts. The profession of nursing represents a larger group of professional people than that of psychiatry, psychology, or social work. The problem of manpower for the mental health field is well known, yet the very people who decry this scarcity demonstrate a tendency to exclude persons who have demonstrable preparation. How can this be? Lay people, who often attribute magical as well as altruistic motives to mental health professionals, would be startled by what would seem to be a simplistic notion. It seems obvious that this group of people should be involved. Sociologists would not be surprised that nurses are not. Hughes states: "The advent of colleague competitors of some new and peculiar type, or by some new route, is likely to arouse anxieties. Colleagues, be it remembered, are also competitors."[1] As nursing emerges and as nurses become better and equally educated, the Triumvirate is challenged and sets up a mutually exclusive, albeit subtle, system. Some of the components of this system include lack of participation in community mental health center planning or, as has occurred on occasion in Colorado, inclusion of nurses who have no mental health background and who would not be the choice of the mental health nursing community, and the exclusion of nurses from staffing the mental health center except in the traditional inpatient setting. It has been interesting to note that only after a community mental health center has been open several years are nurses asked to join the staff. Shouldn't this suffice—to be asked at all, even ex post facto. No, it shouldn't suffice, any more than the exclusion of minority groups should have occurred. As Hughes also states, "The person who is the first of his kind to attain a certain status is often not drawn into the informal brotherhood in which experiences are exchanged, competence built up, and the formal code elaborated and enforced. He thus remains forever a marginal man."[2]

Are nurses the marginal persons of the community mental health center

[1] Hughes, E.: States—dilemmas and contradictions of states. In Coser, L. A., and others, editors: Sociological theory: a book of readings, New York, 1965, The Macmillan Co., p. 370.
[2] *Ibid*, p. 371.

brotherhood (except in providing twenty-four hour care)? If a person is not included in the original grouping he remains forever outside the group. This concept, the Task Force feels, comes as close as any to answering our original question, "If we're so great, how come we have to fight like mad to get into the current community mental health scene?" This concept answers, perhaps, why nurses are not now a part of the scene or are having to fight to be, but the question left unanswered is, "Why weren't nurses part of the original grouping or Grand Triumvirate?" There are many facets of this question that are not answered by defining the pecking order or the marginal man. We feel some answers may be found in looking back at some of the ideas presented to us by other disciplines in addition to our own.

The stereotype

If we could draw a picture of the worst things various disciplines said about a nurse, this is how she would look. She would be found in an institutional setting wearing a white uniform and hiding behind the doctor. She would be holding in one hand a bed pan and in the other a baseball bat. Color her face businesslike. Put few books on her shelf, for she is functionally illiterate, hang a copy of a Nurse Practice Act on her wall and a poster from the social workers saying, "Freud Wants You."

The stereotype emerges with the nurse being a mixture of dependency, passivity, aggressiveness, controlling behavior and is, above all, inadequately educated. In addition to the "bad" stereotype, there was the "good" stereotype. This nurse would be found in the neighborhood, wearing a blue uniform trying to solve the worst problems imaginable, which were graciously given to her by the other members of the community mental health team.

The trouble with stereotypes is that they give a limited, inaccurate picture. Neither of these stereotypes would be particularly valid in describing an individual nurse, and yet each of them contains a part of the truth. The sad fact is that each stereotype has the effect of saying that the nurse is not needed on the mental health team, either in the hospital or in the community.

An even greater disadvantage of stereotyping is that if distance is maintained, the stereotype becomes self-perpetuating, and there is no opportunity for the image to be challenged. However unflattering the stereotypes presented may be, they were not the most frustrating reaction we had. The Task Force unanimously awards the prize for the put-down of the year to the panel member, whose discipline will not be identified, who exhibited an incomparable brand of total indifference. There was no basis for dialogue with this person, and the encounter left us with a feeling of dismay.

The X and the "it" factors

At least one member of nearly every panel mentioned that they were unable to stereotype what was variously called the "it" factor, the something special, or the X factor. Whatever "it" was, though, it was viewed positively. "It" was often proposed as the rationale for including the nurse on the community mental health center team, and as such deserves further exploration.

The nurse clinicians spent a great deal of time discussing the X factor. They felt this factor was made up of the medical and eclectic nature of the educational background of the nurse, the "something holy" or ethics a nurse is taught, her pragmatism, and her orientation to helping. For the Task Force, the term "educated caring" comes the closest to defining concisely what the nurses were calling the X factor.

The panel of psychologists called the uniqueness in the nurse's role "it." While they couldn't define "it," they felt it was made up of (1) a unique relationship with the poor, (2) a degree of closeness and intimacy with patients in the nurse's function that was not tolerated by other professionals, (3) the ability to deal with intimate basic functions that might concern the patient, (4) her practical orientation toward the problem the patient might be having, and (5) *a concern about patients that was somewhat different from the kind of concern other professionals have.*

This concern, or lack of it, that has been noted in the products of nursing and other health education programs is the humanistic concept that can't be held in your hand, but you know "it" when it's present, and when it's not you're experienced as less of a person. Nursing educators take note! This is the concept around which a body of knowledge, not just a set of experiences, can be built. The members of the Task Force do not purport to be experts in the area of curriculum development and are looking to the expertise of the educators in this area. We would, however, like to contribute some of our ideas in this regard. It seems that nursing education is on the right track in providing a liberal arts background. Philosophy, religion, art, and other humanities as well as the basic sciences all contribute to an understanding of the individual. In nursing education this liberal arts background must be blended with technical skills and a greater depth of knowledge in the life sciences. It seems imperative, from what the Task Force has heard, that nursing education demonstrate the ability to produce a practitioner who can blend the humanistic concept with technical skill in understanding wellness as well as the emotional illness of individuals and families. It also is important that the practitioner not be left holding her skills bag but that some means be found by educators and others to continually inform other disciplines and the consumer public that the nurse is thus prepared.

Intraprofessional sparring

Nursing education, or lack of it, was given considerable discussion by all disciplines, including nursing. The statements ranged from "you're getting too much," to "are you getting any at all?" What, where, why, direct patient care versus management, too much, too little—it was a kaleidoscopic collection of statements and questions. We would concede that there are reasons for this confusion.

In the early days of nursing, service and education were one entity. The director of nursing was director both of nursing service and education. Needs of service were closely correlated with the education provided.

As practitioners became upwardly mobile and emphasis was given to nursing education, demands became so heavy that the responsibilities for service and education were separated. Positions in nursing education became the status occupation for practitioners. Nurse educators with advanced preparation constituted an elite corps, and there was a concomitant lessening of rapport between service and education.

Unlike the medical profession, which subscribed to the philosophy of using physicians in active practice as medical educators, there was in nursing an almost complete abdication by nurse faculty from involvement in nursing service. The paucity of nurses with higher degrees caused the siphoning off of those most qualified into nursing education. Salaries for nurse educators were higher than for comparable responsibilities in nursing service, and the potential for career advancement in nursing appeared to be priarily in education.

Within the service area itself, another division was occurring. It became apparent that advancement in institutional nursing could come only through administrative positions, not clinical excellence. Thus, the nurse closest to the patient was at the lowest level in the nursing hierarchy, while those most remote from the patient were at the top of the hierarchical structure. In recent years there has been a gradual shift occurring as many master's prepared nurses enter the clinical field. It is no longer as true as in the past that the best prepared nurse is the farthest from the patient. What provided the impetus for this shift is difficult to identify. It may have been a desire on the part of nurses to return to the humanistic values in nursing and to the bedside. What "bedside" really means is a closeness to individuals and families. Many of the disciplines, including the nursing administrators, seemed to be asking that a balance be found in teaching direct patient care concepts and concepts of organizational structure and management skills. One nurse educator proposed that it might not be a bad idea for baccalaureate student nurses to have experience on evening and night shifts as a means of testing their management skills.

Nursing may not be able to have its cake and eat it, too. It may not be possible for us all to be Libras and find and maintain the balance, but it's worth pondering. Certainly, nursing service and nursing education ought to be able to get together and forget the old battles. One encouraging sign for the future is the certification plan of the American Nurses' Association, using clinical specialty boards to establish criteria and examine credentials. This may result in a colleague relationship between those in service and education.

If the clinical specialist is also compensated for expertise, some of the divisive factors causing the rupture may be eliminated.

The dynamic duo

The pairing of inpatient setting and medication was heard so often that the Task Force dubbed it the "dynamic duo." Our thought was that it was a little like hearing the name "Batman" and immediately associating it with "Robin." These two areas, medication and inpatient service, were usually associated positively as a specialty area of the nurse; whether nurses feel that way about the areas is questionable.

The wisdom of offering medication and functioning on an inpatient setting as a place for the nurse to hang her cap, is debatable; it may be like throwing a boomerang. If what the other disciplines told us is true, all members of the mental health team will share knowledge of medication and its effects and side effects. In addition, giving medication on inpatient units is becoming automated to the point that a nonprofessional may soon be dispensing the drugs. As to the area of managing an inpatient unit, this too may be thin ice. As hospital costs continue to skyrocket, more patients will be cared for in less expensive extended care facilities or in their homes. The need for staff on twenty-four hour units may, in time, dwindle. The dynamic duo is, in fact, not very dynamic and offers very little challenge.

The dumping syndrome

The so-called dumping syndrome has been given considerable discussion already in previous chapters of this book. However, the Task Force would like to make a few final observations about the "dump." The dump is a place where people bring things they no longer want. In mental health or medical parlance, to "dump" means to get rid of an undesirable patient or task. To psychiatric and public health nurses, it frequently means getting the chronic or otherwise undesirable patients nobody else wants.

In truth it is difficult to determine how the dumping syndrome vis-à-vis nurses began. Did nurses originally choose the sicker, more chronic patients? The social worker panelists indicated they did. They said that nurses seem more comfortable with the sicker patients and that as the patient becomes better, the nurse gets uncomfortable and finds somebody to deal with his wellness. The nurse clinicians, on the other hand, felt they were given the chronic patient because no one else wanted them. Whether nurses choose and are more comfortable with illness than wellness or whether they receive undesirable patients because both the nurses and patients are low in status may be a question locked in the proverbial sphinx. The Task Force speculates, however, that the "dump" is a little of both.

We also propose that nurses and the entire mental health team take a fresh look at the so-called dump. Perhaps as one of the nurse clinicians suggested, the nurse is better able to deal with the chronic patient because of her ability to be satisfied with helping and less tangible results rather than curing. It was also pointed out by panelists of other disciplines that the nurse is more practical and able to meet the patient where he is. If these things are true of the nurse then she has a responsibility to teach this skill to other members of the team. To strongly emphasize a point previously made, the chronic patient is a particular problem for community mental health centers because the care of *all* patients within their own community was the mandate under which funds were first made available in 1963. The chronic patient *must* be viewed as a challenge by the entire team.

Adam and Eve

The dominant-submissive aspects of male-female relationships seem as old as Adam and Eve. The passivity attributed to nurses seems equally ancient. While for years we have believed that the problems of the profession were "nursing" problems, it is increasingly evident that the problems are in reality those of females functioning in a male-oriented society. The difficulty of functioning as a female in a male-oriented society has taken its toll within the professional organization. Women, for centuries relegated to a secondary position, exhibit those characteristics to which their sex has conditioned them. There has been an overwhelming inclination to deal with trivialities and ignore broader issues. An almost fanatical insistence on representation from every segment of the nursing profession has resulted in little representation of any kind. The in-fighting among those seeking recognition is a natural outgrowth of the female's vying for male attention. When disputes between members over issues occur, behavior in the ensuing years resembles the saga of the Hatfields and McCoys. Witness the raging battle over the American Nurses' Association position paper, which continues unremittingly five years after its issuance. One despairs that the profession can rise above these characteristics until women in our culture can assume a partnership relationship with men in place of the master-sex symbol system which presently exists.

The Task Force has given these issues a great deal of thought, the passivity attributed to and demonstrated by nurses and the problems of a female operating in a male oriented society, and find they are part and parcel of each other. Speaking to this particular circumstance, the majority of members of the nursing profession are female, and the majority of members of the medical profession are male. Each has learned behavior which society deems fitting for their particular sex. From this relationship has sprung the famous or infamous doctor-nurse game[3] with all its attendant problems. Many nurses and doctors place a great deal of importance on the doctor-nurse game and

---

[3] Stein, L.: The doctor-nurse game, Archives of General Psychiatry **16**:696–703, June 1967.

being able to play it well. They have missed Dr. Stein's point that it is inhibitory, stifling, and dangerous. Nurses often do not or are not allowed to voice their conclusions in a forthright manner, almost as if there were a course in nursing school called Double Talk—the real name of that game is "observation." That nurses observe but do not diagnose is consistently a part of nursing education and has further been legitimized by restrictive nurse practice acts.

Another aspect of the male-female issue has been identified in a previous chapter of the book and is worthy of reiteration. It may well be that, as cited in Chapter 2, women have for centuries been relegated an inferior role in society and, worst of all, have come to believe in their own inferiority. It is obvious that many nurses have come to believe in their own inferiority as women and consequently as nurses. The propensity of the nursing profession to pursue group consensus, nearly to the point of fanaticism, may be another outgrowth of male-female related issues.

The very structure of the professional organization reflects the female orientation of its members. Unlike other similar organizations in which election of officers and boards is accomplished by placing in nomination the name of the candidate for each office and voting unanimously to accept the ballot, the American Nurses' Association ballot provides a minimum of two candidates for each office, and is open for nominations from the floor of the House of Delegates. The practice is polarizing, devisive, expensive, time consuming, and eliminates as potential leaders those who find such an approach distasteful. Can nursing afford to conduct itself like a political entity, or is it time to rise above internal power politics and address itself to the goals of the profession? Since women have been manipulated into a position which prevents them from competing with men on equal grounds, does it make sense to relieve those frustrations by competing with each other? It would appear that the energy devoted to this game might be used more constructively. It appears to the Task Force that "group consensus" and the "democratic process" may be euphemisms for devisive, personal political struggles. A more constructive and real use of the democratic process might be to ensure broad representation on committees designed to resolve problems and issues that affect the group and do, indeed, require some consensus. It is unfortunate that consensus has too often fostered in the nursing profession, restriction, lack of movement (because everyone has to move at once), and has stifled initiative and enthusiasm which lead to change.

PART FIVE
In Trouble Again

Chapter Twelve

PUT IT ALL TOGETHER AGAIN—1983

In this chapter we will attempt to address the major issues raised by the panelists in 1970 and discuss what seems to us to have happened in the last twelve years. We have not reinterviewed enough people from each discipline to do an updated chapter for each one. However, we have accumulated, among the three of us, enough steam on some of the issues to give them another blast, at least a paragraph or two for each discipline.

Psychiatrists: A peek over the pile

The 1970, interviewed psychiatrists were disturbing because of what we, the authors, believed was their limited view of the role of the nurse in community mental health centers. Our discussions with and about the psychiatrists led us to consider the origins and impact of the doctor-nurse game in some detail. We said then that the doctor-nurse game was based on sexist stereotypes, was part and parcel of an authoritarian hierarchical medical model and worked to the detriment of good patient care. We also reported the codependent nature of the relationship and predicted on some glorious day in the future that community mental health centers would be Camelotian indeed with justice and liberty for all, Amen. We were street wise enough to hedge our bet a little, though, and wondered, without wanting to believe it, if the system were not more rigid than it appeared and would not easily give way to an independent, assertive newcomer, the psychiatric nurse. Our hedge is more true today than our wish. Psychiatrists continue to have disturbingly limited views of the role of the nurse, in most instances considering the nurse a semi professional or heaven forbid, a mere physician extender. We have updated examples of responses to masters prepared nurse clinicians which run something like this; this is a true story as told to the authors.

> "Once, during four weeks of a patient's hospitalization I had repeatedly urged the admitting psychiatrist to reconsider his diagnosis of paranoid schizophrenia in favor of manic depressive illness. He had not done so until one day, four weeks later, he called me to say, as if it were a brand new idea, "you know, I really think Mr. _____ is a manic depressive." A long pause on my end of the line ensued. "You thought he might be manic didn't you?" he said slowly. He quickly discounted my early diagnosis by attributing it to the increased time I had allegedly spent with the patient.

It's enough to make one permanently dislocate their TM joints isn't it? There is another true story we want to share for its classic beauty and then we'll move on and give your TM joints (and ours) a rest.

"On a separate occasion, while doing off-hours of crisis work, I was requested to evaluate a delusional, violent patient. After evaluating the patient with his family and arranging for a mental health hold, I staffed the case with two residents at the admitting hopsital. The residents, at the end of my report, asked why I had reached the diagnosis I had. I explained the rationale, to which they nodded agreement. One then asked me, "Did you say you were a nurse?" "Yes," I replied, "Why do you ask?" He said, "Because that was an excellent evaluation."

One of the points this particular nurse clinician made is that, too often, nurses are yet satisfied with whatever crumbs and faint praise they get from psychiatrists instead of expecting respect for their clinical judgments as a matter of course. However, the doctor-nurse game has been attenuated somewhat in the last twelve years by the Women's Movement and there does seem to be some light showing at the end of the tunnel on this issue.

The light only shines though for those who have been fortunate enough to get in and hang on to their positions during these tough economic times. Nurses were often the last hired and first fired while predominantly male, higher ranked, and more expensive positions emerged unscathed. So, sexist attitudes continue to affect nurses in the '80's and are perhaps even more blatant as the economy becomes the predominant issue. We won't even bore you, the readers, with all the statistics about percentage of females in the work force, the wide differences in salary for men and women, numbers of female heads of household, job classifications based on sex not responsibility; no, we know that you know the system.

The mental health centers and the psychiatrists therein who occupied positions of power were the group we perhaps hoped to influence most twelve years ago. We did not foresee the dramatic exodus of psychiatrists from the public to the private sector. We have considered some of the reasons for the psychiatrists' decampment and have one or two more stories to tell. Psychiatrists were at the top of the pile in 1971. In June, 1982 their position had changed somewhat. "Where did we go wrong?", lamented one chief psychiatrist. He said, "I think it was when we started to play volleyball with the staff and patients in the therapeutic communities. I hated volley ball in the first place," he continued, "and I never thought it really helped anybody. The social workers would always get upset with me though when I brought it up." Then he delivered the coup de grace which was . . . "It was then (when the social workers were confronting him we presume) that the nurse would come to my side" (to defend him, poor dear and so dependent). Again, the physician saw the alliance with the nurse as being different in character from other members of the team and definitely more comforting. It is so hard to get good help these days, isn't it? But lest we trash the alliance between doctors and nurses completely, let us say that we think it has aspects of value, as well. All we would wish for is a relationship of shared respect, rather than mutual dependence. The authors think that the democratization of community mental health centers and so-called therapeutic communities was more than many psychiatrists could take. We also think there was a false egalitarianism that served no one well. There have also been major advances in neurophysiology which have changed the practice of psychiatry, the trend now being to a biological model. This has put the psychiatrist back into the white coat and (thank God) off the volley ball court.

In the intervening years quite a few nurses have had the opportunity to work in positions in the psychiatric emergency room, mental health centers, and in private practice where they had independent decision making, accountability and direct responsibility for the client. Nurses have studied the nature and process of their practice and have made many advances toward independent practice in the hospital setting as well. All these factors have produced some change in the relationship between nurses and psychiatrists. It has produced some serendipitous learning as well and the authors pass it along in a "for what it's worth" vein. In the old doctor-nurse game, nurses learned to be deferential and subservient. At least one of the authors has since learned that that's not the way to get along with the species at all. The real secret is if you're dealing with more than one doctor you have to be a little mean to them. You have to overwhelm them slightly with esoteric, current research findings in order to gain their respect. We say this somewhat, but not entirely, tongue in cheek. Nurses, we think, are still too prone to be relieving everybody's anxieties which is not, if you observe their behavior, the way doctors learn. Doctors learn in a battleground of one upsmanship; watch Grand Rounds sometime or how doctors tease each other if you doubt the truth of this. One psychiatrist, who shall remain anonymous for obvious reasons of safety, imparted this secret knowledge to one of the authors. This disbelieving nurse has put the secret to the test and found it remarkably useful.

So, we will leave the beleaguered, but richly reimbursed, psychiatrist for another ten years perhaps. Nurses, we think, are a little wiser, more confident, somewhat more respected and certainly less willing to play the old doctor-nurse game.

Psychologists: The truth will out

We suspected, in 1970, that the glorification of the non-pursuit of degrees by the psychologists, all of whom had Ph.D.'s you will recall, was somehow false. Twelve years later we have some evidence that our suspicions were well founded. Not only did nurses ignore the psychologists' probably well-intentioned advice, but psychologists ignored it, too. They seemed in fact in the '80's not to look kindly upon the master's level psychologist, or on certain kinds of doctoral degrees as well. In order to enter the brotherhood, and a highly lucrative one it is these days, one must not only possess a doctorate in psychology, but it must be a doctorate in clinical psychology as well. No more Ed. Psych degrees will do. What happened to romping through the grassroots together anyway? Oh well, we as nurses have had our bouts with certification and third party payments and who is qualified to do what, so perhaps we have some sympathy for the psychologists' increasingly stringent rules; some, but not much, for psychologists have been less than helpful to nurses in some Eastern seaboard states where nurses were seeking inclusion in the state's laws governing third party payments. Nurses from these states reported fierce opposition from psychologists. For shame. And here we thought we were going to tiptoe through the tulips together. Well, one more hope bites the dust. Most of us didn't really believe we had true respect from the panel of psychologists in the '70's, but we didn't count on their total lack of support and active opposition in state after state as nurses fought for recognition.

We guess the lesson is, that all was well as long as there was enough pie for everyone; they made more than we did anyway. But as more and more people in all mental health disciplines entered the private sector things turned a little ugly. Nurses who have fought some of those guerrilla battles have something to teach the rest of us about obtaining and maintaining power. We had best listen.

Licensed psychiatric technicians—The kick became a field goal

In Colorado, in 1983, Licensed Psychiatric Technicians are employed only in state run psychiatric and mental retardation facilities and their total number has diminished. There is a nine month training program offered at two community colleges in the state and licensure is still offered via the state nursing board for graduates of the certification program in Colorado or from out of state.

Mental Health Worker is the job title that most persons who work in community mental health centers are listed under and what many people who were licensed technicians have become. These people have either a two-year degree in the Human Services field or a minimum of a B.S. in Psychology and one year of experience. They are found doing bits and pieces of everything as shown in a breakdown of the functional survey conducted by the Colorado Division of Mental Health in 1981.[1]

One mental health worker who works in a private psychiatric hospital also has his own active private practice in marital counseling. He sees nurses as good but narrow in role and functioning as primarily custodial and Ratched-like.* This person in his discussion with one of the authors said "I believe the whole mental health system is built to feed itself. Everyone is out to keep

---

[1] Colorado Division of Mental Health Report, 1981.
* From *One Flew Over the Cuckoo's Nest.*

patients in some dependent relationship. What will really rock the boat is when the public wises up and learns that most of them can get well in other ways like transcendental meditation, yoga and biofeedback. The people that really need the help are the chronically ill patients. I believe in holistic health and all that, but there are the bipolar depressed people, other affective disorders and drug addictions. These illnesses take a whole different treatment and a bunch of research. I'm really turned off to keeping so many people dependent when we could be doing so much more." Who could disagree? We wouldn't.

Another mental health worker said "the term 'technician' was degrading, and nursing was a big supporter as we tramped off to community colleges to get Associate Arts Degrees." So the kick from behind did become a field goal now; as one mental health worker stated, "In my opinion, mental health workers run the centers." In 1971 we identified the indigenous worker as being one of the under utilized sources of manpower. We could have saved ourselves the worry. In 1981 indigenous workers, if we accept the current mental health workers as indigenous, comprise fifty-seven percent of the staff of mental health centers in Colorado.[2] We, the authors, think there is much danger for patients in a system that allows itself to compromise the balance between personnel who have specific and identifiable bodies of knowledge and those who do not; witness conditions in many nursing homes. We think, still, that a combination of social action, primary prevention and treatment of illness is the only sane model for quality services.

Social workers: They've scored but can they win?

1983 seems to have the Social Workers less concerned about whether psychiatric nurses know Freudian theory though the turf battle still exists. Perhaps the social workers have less to worry about than they did 12 years ago because if indeed there was a battle (we believe there was, and is) the social workers may have won. They, at least in Colorado, have the same manpower percentages as nurses but they have moved into higher level administrative positions in mental health. Today multiple theoretical frameworks dominate psychiatric practice so less is heard about Freud. Social work has had problems in credentialing but it seems to have weathered this better than nurses have. Perhaps it is because they are fewer in number and have you noticed . . . they aren't all female. In fact in Colorado most seem to be well-established in their roles. As one social worker stated, "I worked in community mental health centers for ten years, both in Colorado and New York. It had its satisfactions primarily because you were involved in therapy and worked together as a team. Frankly, I didn't know what most people's

---

[2] *Ibid.*

backgrounds were. I knew I was paid more than some because I have a Master's degree, but other than that we all did a bit of everything. I don't remember turf troubles; we didn't dispense medicines in the Center *so I guess nurses didn't have much of a role.*" Ouch—the song may be ended but the medicine lingers on.

In 1970 the panelists we interviewed believed that social workers cared for the "well" and nurses for the "sick." The public health nurse was identified as a quasi member of the mental health team. The public health nurse (the quasi member) cared for chronic mentally ill patients who needed follow-up on medications. In the past decade this has changed, it has been personnel from mental health centers who are working with the chronic patients. Public health/community health nurses seem to have a diminished role in mental health per se. But changes in funding may see a shift back to an increase in the public health nurse's involvement in mental health as home health options become broader. The social workers who were already comfortable with this role of the nurse should have little problem with that unless, of course, they want it for themselves. That is not an impossibility as social workers have, at least in Colorado, via legislative funding, assumed much of the case management of many Home Health patients as an alternative to the nursing home program called Senate Bill 38 and 138. Community Health Nursing fought a battle over this one and lost. This process may be something we need to closely scrutinize. Social workers in general have somewhat less unique characteristics than other disciplines. They lack the physiological or medical knowledge of psychiatrists and nurses and the research knowledge base of *some* psychologists. Social workers' greatest contribution seems to be in bridging gaps, that is the transitional stages in a health-illness continuum; with an emphasis on family support and community networks. And, bridging the gaps was not financially a high priority . . . so many social workers headed for private practice.

A look at the yellow pages of the Denver phone directory yields fascinating information when contrasting psychiatric nurses and social workers. For instance, social workers are identified as doing all kinds of psychiatric private practice, but nurses, on the other hand, don't identify themselves as "nurses." They are also far out-numbered by social workers in private practice. It appears as though we must take our nurse's caps off to the social workers because they seem to be moving upward both in private practice and in mental health facilities.

Nurses view their world

Like it or not . . . it's a small world after all . . . a world of laughter and a world of tears . . . a world of hope and a world of fears . . . (to paraphrase Walt Disney's "It's a Small World") and to the nurse of 1983 quite a changed world than we found in 1971. Three separate 'worlds' of nursing were sources for the chapters on nursing in the first edition: the clinicians, the educators, and the administrators. Because the educators seemed to "get it" from both the clinician and the administrator, we chose to find out about them first. How have the ivory tower idealists fared during the decade? First, we were surprised to find a good number of them no longer hiding out in the dusty stacks of libraries polishing up their latest theory of nursing. Instead they had donned white coats of the nurse practitioner, or were sitting on hospital boards deciding the wisdom of opening or closing a treatment unit. Clearly the small world of academe had a minor explosion. From whence, pray tell, did the enlightenment come? Remember how the 1971 educators spoke only of passive students that had to be directly questioned about their clinical practice? Somewhere in their pressured lives to publish or perish, to climb the academic ladder to heaven called Tenure, 'patient' had become a foreign word and clinical practice a foreign land. Administrators and clinicians (as well as the other disciplines) in 1971 cast disparaging remarks about the negative result of being socialized in the nunnery/military school environment of the SON (School of Nursing). Creativity and cunning supposedly were squelched from the students' bones as they entered the hallowed halls of professional education.

Yes, certainly some enlightenment came from the negative criticism. Nurse educators found themselves so far out on a limb that E.T.'s phone couldn't even reach them. Some educators fortunately or unfortunately, were lopped off because of their own irrelevance while other educators sat up and took notice, thankfully before it was too late.

Strange but meaningful working relationships between the educator-clinician, the clinician-educator and the administrator-educator began. Several schools of nursing (U. of Rochester, U. of Wisconsin, U. of Washington, U. of Colorado, U. of California, San Francisco—*to name but a few*) have developed collaborative clinician roles for nurse educators. Nurse administrators in many university settings now have legitimate professorial rank and status.

In addition to uniting into a closer, smaller world, nurse educators have been far more active in their own clinical roles. Striving for promotion no longer could be based on pure academic achievement but vitae were also scrutinized for bits of evidence of community service and clinical practice. Consequently nurse educators, being squeezed by the same financial crunch as other academicians, needed to legitimize their being. The push for certification came as a backlash to the rapid expansion of the alternative health care provider. One couldn't distinguish one legitimate guru from another! The push toward certification occurred during the first part of the decade (much as we had predicted). What did certification mean to nurse educators and to all of nursing? Besides measuring knowledge in a specialized area, certification demanded that certifiable nurses have actual patient or client contact. No ivory tower or text book alone would suffice. Consequently in the '70's large numbers of faculty returned to clinical laboratories to get prepared as 'nurse practitioners.' (We would like to say that the nurse practitioner program was first begun under the direction of Dr. Loretta Ford, at the University of Colorado. She is presently Dean of the School of Nursing, University of Rochester). Psychiatric nursing faculties claimed that at the graduate level they always prepared practitioners. However, numerous psychiatric-mental health nursing faculty members became actively engaged in part-time clinical practice. Thus, the push toward certification succeeded in breaking down, a bit, the ivory tower and sometimes released a long-forgotten captive princess.

Captive princesses always seemed fragile and unfulfilled in fairy tales unless some daring suitor climbed the treacherous wall or kissed the curse away. Perhaps the push out of the captive cell has only begun but those princesses who have escaped tell tales of how invigorating it is to be "free." Surprisingly educators now in some type of clinical practice like it! As one who directs a rural clinic said, "I really look forward to Tuesdays away from the School. I'm exhausted after seeing twenty or so kids, but it's so meaningful." Another, who maintains a part-time position in a group practice of psychiatric nurse clinicians said, "No one could have told me before that I could *both* teach and practice. Not only do I teach better, but I practice better. Students say I'm more alive and spontaneous. They, in turn, give me great ideas about some tough clinical problems." An associate dean in a large university hospital said, "Maintaining a joint practice in the hospital is demanding—yet it has given faculty something we've fought for for years—credibility and visibility. I think we're more sensitive to staffing problems and I hope we've added to the quality of care. We have, as nurses, assumed what is rightfully ours . . . the shared responsibility for good clinical care. Somewhere along the way to professionalism we lost territory when Schools of Nursing faculty became so separated from clinical practice."

Another reason for a closer relationship between nursing education and clinical practice has come from a shift in research funding. In the late '70's clinically based practical research was the only type being funded. Nurse researchers aren't dumb! If you want a high priority number you had better research what is being supported. Competition for the very limited number of research grants increased the need for nurse educators to get with it in a clinical setting for as one faculty member said, "Before I re-entered clinical practice I could not think of a research proposal; now, as a result of being in practice, ideas are popping out every minute. I see so many possibilities for research that I never saw before . . . I can really be a resource for students struggling for master's and doctoral topics for research."

In spite of closer working relationships much still remains controversial. In particular disenchantment over the integrated curriculum has spread nationally. "The idea of integrating mental health concepts into all aspects of nursing was a critical step and we mustn't forget the progress we have made," said one nursing leader. "However", she continued, "teaching integrated mental health concepts doesn't go too far when a student is working with an acutely psychotic person or with chronic psychoses. We need desperately to re-establish strong guidelines and standards for educating undergraduate students in mental illness." Education of the baccalaureate level nurse in psychiatric care . . . not merely integrated mental health concepts . . . is a high priority in the future for the Nursing Division of NIMH. The same can be said for community-public health nursing.

Contrary to the so-called good advice of the 1971 psychologists, nurses have continued to go back to school for higher education. For instance there was an increase in master's programs—to 142 in 1981, a gradual decrease in full-time enrollment, and an increased graduation rate.[3] We salute the nurse educators who have taken up the challenge and re-entered the real world of nursing practice.

Nurse administrators—Powwow redefined

The Nurse Administrators in the '71 book met with the nurse educators and we extrapolated their comments. For this book no one met with anyone and we did not interview nurse administrators. Since two of us are administrators we will attempt to deal with the '83 issues.

The Nurse Practice Acts maligned in '71 have changed in many states and appear to not be the kind that "box in" but rather make different levels of practice possible. The nurse practitioner and the nurse clinician will presumably be legally covered by the Acts to practice. These new Practice Acts will undoubtedly be tested in the courts particularly in the areas of prescriptive privileges. Third party payments are being made more possible by nurses going to state legislation to lobby for inclusion in insurance payments due to the Acts being modernized to reflect current practice.

In the social worker 1971 chapter, there was concern about services being duplicated by public health nurses and the mental health center; we found duplication of functions was less of a concern in the '70's as mental health centers were the major providers. However, as we predicted in 1971, and our crystal ball keeps saying the same thing, that public health nurses (either in public health agencies or home health agencies) will again resume the major mental health service role. That is unless other mental health workers see functioning within communities such as doing well oldster groups in public health programs or making home mental health follow-ups, etc. as being economically lucrative or feasible. Do not forget how economics dictates the movement of the so-called health care system.

---

[3] Vaughn, J. Educational Preparation for Nursing, 1981. Nursing and Health Care, Vol. 3, No. 8, 1982, p. 450.

There is little reason that a public health nurse could not do and probably already does those things for patients/clients/family that keep people healthy mentally and physically. Many nurses come to public health with psychiatric backgrounds and should not be discouraged from functioning particularly with mental health (preferably nurse) consultation available to them. If indeed the mental health centers are on their way out as funding diminishes, public health agencies, as they continue to identify community aggregate needs, will need to build in programs for those in need of mental health services not dealt with by the private sector. In Colorado, interestingly enough, a development worthy of note is the potential coming back together under one agency of public health and mental health. The Mental Health Division of the State Health Department separated over a decade ago when the monies were plentiful in order to establish their own separate programs. Going around in circles makes one's head spin, doesn't it?

Nursing Administrators in 1971 were perhaps more passive-aggressive in their feelings toward educators then they are now. Administrators of nursing service had been saying to educators that clinical opportunities would be provided to students if the agency or institution got something in return such as input into curricula or continuing educational programs for the staff as well as adjunctive faculty appointments. In Colorado, for the last year at least one specialty area—community health, has had meetings of University faculties and health department nursing service administrators. These meetings have been to share ideas and to give mutual input. This is most positive and again was something that was done years ago but faded into the sunset. We believe it's important and that the sun continues to shine on every effort to have nursing educators and nursing administrators work together.

One other positive parenthetical note is that nurse administrators, under the auspices of ANA, have developed their own certification process. Certification brings administrators closer to the current state of the Art in nursing.

The psychiatric nurse clinician—1983 style

Nostalgia and some sadness were the feelings of the authors as we reread the 1971 material on psychiatric nurse specialists. We didn't know it then, in Colorado, but that time was the Camelot for master's prepared nurses in the community mental health center. A nurse hired to do full time clinical research and publication, can you believe that? It is also with nostalgia that the authors remember the vitality, the intelligence and the humor of that group of panelists. They were wonderful. They were the group that wrestled "it", the special quality or uniqueness of the nurses' role, to the mat. They gave us, the whole field of psychiatric-mental health nursing, the x-factor, that educated caring, that "something holy" that makes the nurses relationship to the patient/client unique. Whole conferences, the yearly symposia of Dr. Madeleine Leininger on Caring for example, are now devoted to defining and refining this concept.

Research priorities in the late 1970's and early 1980's clearly shifted toward clinical concerns and "care." We also remember, though, the concept of "care, cure, coordination" (Remember that?) When this definition of nursing (as adopted by the American Nurses Association in 1964) was introduced to the panel everyone nearly choked. "Ick," they said. "It does not compute," they said. But "it" kept bothering everyone and the discussion then returned to the issue until definition and a sense of closure was reached. It was a good time in nursing, we think.

So much has changed in the last twleve years. Instead of being found in a community mental health center as a member of the Big Four, the 1983 style nurse clinician may be found in full-time private practice earning as much as $40,000 to $50,000 a year. We realize that relatively few private nurse clinicians are earning this much, but some are. In 1970 none were. In 1970 the frontier was the psychiatric emergency room team staffed entirely by nurses and the community mental health center outpatient team. In 1983 the frontier is, we think, private practice; that too shall fade and be replaced by—what— the State Hospital? Stranger things have happened. For now with this book, though, we'll stick to the present and draw a new picture of the psychiatric nurse. Picture this nurse in private practice with three other clinicians each of whom have $40,000 to $50,000 a year practices. Most of their clients have good insurance that reimburses at the rate of $50 per hour. Incidentally, this is about the amount charged by those psychotherapists regardless of title or educational preparation. This nurse's private clients come weekly or biweekly for a fifty-minute hour to a well furnished office renting for approximately $1,000 to $2,000 monthly. This nurse is keeping insurance records, buying answering machines, bell boys, and purchasing computer time for billing purposes. It's a whole new bag of tricks that an altruistic professional education didn't anticipate. Instead of a mop or a bedpan the new nurse needs a calculator, DSM III, a journal of court Rulings and Appeals as well as the daily Wall Street Journal. We might add this therapist views her chronic patients as those with full insurance benefits and that she refuses to see Medicare patients. "They only reimburse us at a rate of $12.50 per hour; it's not enough to meet expenses." This situation is not unusual as others we interviewed expressed many of the same views; caught in the rat race of entrepreneurship, the nurses have to do what others in private practice have done, look at costs and benefits and become hard-nosed business people. "Social reform and concern is great," one said, "but it better not hit my pocket book." This composite nurse in private practice lists chief concerns for continuing education, as: "how to get third party reimbursements," "how to handle estates of deceased" and "how to publicize or attract and keep clientele." When this nurse is asked if the private therapy route meets the social needs of the community such as reaching the poor, the young, and the old, the reply is filled with conflict. She may say, "I worry about that a lot, but I believe we in private practice are seeing chronic patients; it's the community mental health centers that care for the crises."

We wonder, though, what will happen to those chronically mentally ill patients presently being seen in the private sector now that insurance coverage for those conditions has been cut so drastically. There is a real dilemma here that needs to be addressed. With greater numbers of nurses entering private practice, though not nearly in the numbers of other professions, we have to take a look at the needs of society and the fact that health care in this country is big business. David Osborne writing in Harper's, September, 1982, in "Rich Doctors, Poor Nurses," says what others have also noted, that the free market system doesn't exist in the health care sector.[4] Physicians, through the AMA, have pushed out the competition and as a result consumers have little choice. Third party payments further defeat any motivation for competitive pricing. Nurses, as long as the price fixing is in effect, are free to charge the going rate of $50–$150 an hour. We wonder though if such a system really serves the needs of society. What about using some of our political clout to break the system and help bring costs for health care within reach of the average person. Is any professional really worth that much money? We think the amount of money most physicians and hospitals make in this country is obscene. The dilemma is, how can nurses reap their fair share of the money to be made without adding to this greedy system? We think perhaps the only way to do this is to break down the strangle hold physicians have on the cost of service. We could join perhaps in class action suits with other disciplines, notably psychologists and social workers, against the AMA. Such a suit was recently brought, in fact, by psychologists in Oklahoma. However, please do not construe this with any mystical ambivalence about pay. Nurses still have a long way to go before they are, as a group, in any danger of entering the big leagues in salary. A comparison of modal salaries of full time private sector professionals[5] compiled by the state of Colorado for 1979 shows the following:

Discipline	Modal Salary, 1979, Priv. Sector
Psychiatrist	$50,000–74,999
Psychologist	30,000–39,999
Nurse	15,000–19,999
Social Worker	15,000–19,999

Nurses as a group, during the 1970's and 1980's, have profited from increased unionism, collective bargaining and, let's face it, strikes. Compare

---

[4] Osborne, D. Rich Doctors, Poor Nurses. Harper's, September, 1982, pp. 11.
[5] Colorado Private Sector Mental Health Survey, 1980. Mental Health Association of Colorado, 1981, p. 15.

the salary figures above with those compiled in 1969.[6] Note: these salaries are for the public sector so for psychiatrists at least we're comparing apples and oranges.

Discipline	Modal Salary, 1969, Pub. Sector
Psychiatrist	$21,600
Psychologist	13,776
Social Worker	10,440
Nurse	7,236

At least we've made it into a five figure salary range in the last twelve years. The economic gain of nurses in Colorado since 1969 is about 232% in comparison to social workers' 144%. However, these figures are for the public sector and are probably one good reason that there is a full page in the Denver telephone books yellow pages of social worker listings.

In the first chapter we said economics was the bottom line in the defeat of the ERA and that the same factors mitigate against the profession of nursing. We still say that is true. But let's do it better than the others. Let's not let the system get away with painting the higher nurses' salaries as the sole reasons for increases in health care costs.

Many of the nurse clinicians we spoke with were very concerned with social issues. They were outraged at the situation of the "street people," they were concerned about delinquency, violence, drug and alcohol abuse, the borderline patient, the chronically mentally ill and the criminally insane. They were concerned with legal issues concerning patients' rights, commitment laws, and the delicate balance between the right to privacy and freedom of information and the difference between a right as prescribed by law and a need for confidentiality as a condition of treatment. Most of the clinicians with whom we spoke were no longer employed by community mental health centers. One said, "Out here the word is never mentioned." In some sections of the country great debates are raging over the terms 'specialist' versus 'practitioner,' psychiatric versus mental health, the value of prevention versus treatment, holistic and self help groups wage war with the psychobiologists. We think the debates are great; long may they live.

Another change noted in the '80's is that there is such a difference, too, in the quality of nursing publications. Very polished, scientific articles are being written by nurses which one of the authors proudly distributes for the edification of other professionals. Quite a change has taken place, in many respects we think.

At the close of this chapter we would voice the challenge that the debate continue, no more grovelling for pay, please, and at the same time that we

---

[6] Colorado Mental Health Manpower, WICHE, Boulder, Colorado, 1971, p. 23.

work for the betterment of the health care system by whatever means we are able. We found no more mops with this group; no one willing to warm the seat for the doctor and that the whole doctor-nurse game had become less problematic. By and large we are surprised to find ourselves ending this chapter on a more optimistic note than we thought we would. The biggest disappointment was the failure of nurses to break into or influence the community mental health center system in any significant way. However, we have lots of company in the unemployment lines as funding for the centers decreases. The centers, as has been pointed out by some nursing leaders, though, did provide our profession with a model for independent practice that we didn't have before. For that we're grateful; the rest we leave to your imagination.

Chapter Thirteen

TAKING IT APART AGAIN

Now you have come to the last chapter of this new edition. The turmoil of the late '60's was fertile field for our first edition of *Out of Uniform and Into Trouble*. Banning the bra and streaking were then symbols of letting go of old traditions and outmoded restrictions. In nursing many of us did go out of uniform and struggled for a new definition of the nurse's role in community health centers and in other community settings. We squirmed and struggled to be in the mainstream of the triumverate of psychologists, psychiatrists, and social workers; we cursed the fact that we were "marginal" and that others sometimes at best ignored us. We didn't want to "shuffle baby shuffle" any more but rather to march as equals into the sunsets of peace and love. But to be equals we needed to understand (and perhaps plot against) what the Holy Three thought of us and also what the somewhat demeaned licensed psychiatric technicians thought.

It was our belief a decade ago that the vital issues for all health personnel and nurses in particular, whether in general health or mental health settings, were prevention, the role of social action, mental health manpower, and power and how it was used by us and against us. Once again, although we do not pretend to be experts we would like to take one last opportunity to address the issues we feel are vital to the total health system.

The primacy of prevention and the role of social action—or living in a dream world

The model in which most persons in the mental health profession receive their basic education is an illness model. It is more than somewhat ludicrous that the group is called health and its model is illness. Lip service, a service which we are quite adept at delivering, is paid to the primacy of prevention while the actual delivery of services is to illness. There is controversy in the mental health establishment about whether or not primary prevention is a legitimate goal. There is a body of opinion organized around the belief that our society will always produce psychiatric casualties and that the legitimized role as given by the community and perpetuated by the illness model is to care for these casualties in the mental health center. Further, the illness model and the community which supports it have neither given nor allowed for the development of more than scanty tools for primary prevention. It is contended that primary prevention belongs to the education specialist and others outside the mental health establishment. In our social system, we wait for an act of God or legislation to allow people the right to vote, to obtain education, and to receive the best health possible, physical or mental. In the meantime, we have poured funds into the building of edifices and weapons to destroy people in our insane arms race. We then measure success by the number of people that are seen in these buildings who are unable to cope with competition and stress. The primary prevention group has failed too, we believe, by holding that their approach is the only rational approach to mental health and by sitting on their hands feeling persecuted while allowing the buildings to be built. Failure to sell this model or to develop the "clout" in order to do the selling has perpetuated enchantment with the illness model. They then cry, not too silently, for stricter law enforcement and locked wards and locked-in people. Isn't it possible that we can integrate the views of the need for prevention and the realities of some forms of illness and come up with a model for social action that most groups can believe in, support, and sell.

Social action as an entity is left with either youth or minorities as its advocates. In order to attain social action aimed at primary prevention, as well as the care of the inevitable casualties, we would like to propose the dimensions we feel the mental health model must have. This model must incorporate social action as a part of primary prevention as well as caring for the illness component. How to achieve this model or how we get there from here is obviously complex, since this model must be based on an awareness of its place in the total health picture.

It is our feeling that the consistency with which the 1971 panelists referred to the public health model has implications for our belief that it is desirable to incorporate this at some level as a viable preventive model. The image of health and mental health ought to reflect, at one level, an example to society, and at another level, an innovator and proponent of programs whose outcome could mean better physical and mental health for all. It is inconceivable, and yet more true than not, that a coordinated approach to problem solving only exists in a minute way in the current system. We wonder how many persons in the mental health field have become politically involved so that they could influence such efforts as fair housing, equal educational opportunities, social security and sex education, only to mention a few. Yet this is social action and primary prevention. Somehow all of us must find some way to combine all that is good in the illness model and combine it with prevention to form a mental health model.

Nearly all our 1983 respondents said in one way or another that the mental health center movement is dead or dying and that they are in reality mental illness centers. Furthermore, one person stated that the centers failed not only to be health centers, they failed miserably also as illness centers. This nurse clinician said, "If you want to see the outcome of the mental health center movement's drive to deinstitutionalize patients, you should see the street people of New York; you would not believe it; there are thousands of psychotic, organic patients who have been turned out on the streets and they have nothing." This nurse thought that the public, even before Reagonomics became a factor, had been disillusioned by the failure of the mental health centers to provide effective programs for the chronically mentally ill. She also said that in the part of the country she lives in the word mental health centers is "never mentioned." It was almost a spooky experience for the authors of *Out of Uniform* to read what we had said about the possible dangers to the mental health system of isolating itself from the larger health system. We feared then the identity with the aggressor phenomenon. As it turned out, the larger system simply let the minority, mental health centers, do themselves in so to speak. In 1971 we were worried about funding for prevention. Today in 1983 it's difficult to get funding even for illness. As an example, there have been massive cuts in insurance benefits for mental health-psychiatric care. A weak protest has been heard from physicians on the matter of these benefit cuts, but we've heard nothing of a grass roots rebellion against the wiping out of a whole class of health services.

Mental health manpower

We hoped in 1971 that mental health centers would mirror as well as provide models for society. We also secretly hoped that nurses would lead the way as social action innovators combining the best of the illness models with the best of the prevention model to form a mental health model. That did not happen. A Western Interstate Commission of the Higher Education, WICHE survey done during the winter of 1982 had some interesting findings in regard to how nurses view the mental health issues in their community. Two-hundred twenty-nine nurses responded to the questionnaire. These respondents were primarily (40 percent) from the Western States. The other 60 percent represented all of the United States. Thirty-nine percent of the respondents were employed in schools of nursing, 21 percent in general hospitals, 13 percent were in private hospitals, and 6 percent were in community mental health settings. One-eighth of all the nurses were in private practice; the remaining nurses were employed in various governmental settings.[1]

Out of the responses, funding of resources was seen as the major problem facing communities. The federal cutbacks in service were predicted to have severe and long standing detrimental effects. The top clinical concern was around the general issue of violence such as family abuse and rape. Borderline patients were also a major concern. Another broad issue was the area of psychopharmacology and the biochemistry of mental illness. Those clinicians in private practice were primarily interested in reimbursement while clinicians in community mental health centers were distraught by funding cutbacks that would decrease services to the poor. Clinicians working in state institutions ranked care of the chronically ill as the major concern. Private practice cli-

---

[1] Western Interstate Commission for Higher Education, Newsletter, Winter, 1982, pp. 1–5.

nicians also were very concerned about issues in women's health care and in research to determine efficacy of treatment. For faculty, efficacy of treatment and biochemical research were major interests. Indications of an increased trend toward private practice was evidenced of respondents as 50 percent indicated an interest in establishing a private practice. It is interesting to note the specificity of the information they wanted, i.e. opportunities for practice, state regulations, legal issues, record keeping, the politics of lobbying for reimbursement, admitting privileges, advertising and referral sources.[2]

It appears from this study, which is consistent with what we were told by our respondents, that the trend in mental health nursing is toward private practice and other community settings, not into mental health centers. Also, a Colorado public sector, mental health centers, study of percent of time spent by mental health disciplines in various job activities in mental health centers comparison 1969 to 1981 showed that the percent of nurses employed in mental health centers had remained the same. The study showed that the time spent in administration by nurses had decreased by 14 percent while the time spent by social workers in administration had increased by 22 percent.[3,4] Who do you suppose are the new center directors these days? The same study also showed that psychiatrists' numbers had decreased markedly and that psychologists had shifted from administration to clinical work. Clinical work for psychologists was up 54 percent.[5]

Has quality lost its flavor on the bedpost overnight

Quality is a term that is bandied about these days as the raison d'etre for a whole host of issues relating to nursing. We do not disagree that quality is probably the most important argument we have in defending nursing's right to exist. We are concerned that it has been over used to the point it has become meaningless. We would like to try to breathe some new life into the term. The x-factor was something that everyone of the original panels brought up as being the unique factor in nurse-patient relationships. In the first edition of *Out of Uniform* we called it "educated caring." The authors think the x-factor is closely related to quality. We asked one of our respondents in 1982 what she thought had happened to that "something holy" or ethics that a nurse doesn't go in with but comes out with. She said she thought that students come out with a little less of "it." This may be partly a result of changes in nursing education which places less emphasis on tradition, or it may just be a reflection of changes in values in society as a whole. We don't propose that we are experts or have the answers, we just pose the issue as food for thought.

One thing we did hear fairly consistently from our respondents and in

---

[2] *Ibid.*
[3] Colorado Association for Mental Health, 1981.
[4] Colorado Division of Mental Health Report, 1981.
[5] *Ibid.*

meetings across the country was the move to cut clinical practice more and more in both undergraduate and graduate programs in nursing. The authors are well aware that most educators take serious exception to the idea of maintaining, or even, heaven forbid, increasing supervised clinical practice. However, before we get shouted down by the loyal opposition which says it's not needed because of integrated curriculum, we ask that some of you consider that students coming into nursing may still be people who are interested in practical results and who want to have good direct patient care skills. In addition, we think they also want sound theoretical frameworks and a knowledge base from which to practice. The experience of the authors in and out of hospitals as staff and sometimes as patients during the last few years has convinced us that the professional nurse of today does or can give quality patient care. We think that knowledgeable, competent care does make a difference in terms of decreased pain, faster recovery, and infinitely greater patient satisfaction.

We think though, that there is another important element in the quality of patient care, at least in the hospital setting. We think that element is the system within which nursing is practiced. We are sure this comes as no surprise to the nurse-sociologists among us but we wonder how many of you have experienced the difference in the nursing care delivered via the old "functional" system versus the "primary" nursing system. Those of us who had seen both had these experiences. With primary nursing the experience was characterized by being treated with respect, having one's questions answered without the "you'll have to ask the doctor run around," and consideration of pain as a legitimate issue. Functional nursing on the other hand was marked by seeing the nurse only when there was a hassle, fights among staff over whose job was what and general chaos which left staff and patients exhausted. Cheers and strokes to those nurse administrators who continue to fight the battles over needing to deliver patient care by professional nurses in whichever setting patients are found. We need to use our clinical research skills and prove how much better this is for patients.

Here we go again and again and again

Although this may seem an odd change from the issue of quality, we have in the last twelve years developed some more ideas about nursing's fanatical need for consensus. One idea is that decision making is difficult because many of us want everyone to like us. Hence, decisions are hashed and rehashed and sent sideways and up and down in the organization in the search for total agreement. It seems also that if there is a disagreement expressed there is an obsession within the group to resolve the difference. It means that people are really not free to disagree because if they do they're hounded until they agree so that everyone can go home guilt free. In the meantime decision making comes to a halt. We are certainly not suggesting that an attempt not be made to resolve different points of view but must there be the endless search for total agreement? We would like to see a higher tolerance for conflict. We think the endless search for consensus is one reason for energy's being used up and the relative powerlessness of professional nursing organizations. It will be interesting to see if ANA's recent structural change gives us more power to deal with specific issues.

"General Hospital," "Nurse" or MASH

An important reflection of power or powerlessness is image. In our first study, which you have now read, we discussed our image as nurses and that we needed to do something about the stereotypes people have in their mind when the word "nurse" is used. Our findings 12 years later led us to believe we've still got a long, long way to go. From our discussions and interviews we find a strange image of nursing that emerges as a cross between a Joan Crawford and a Mother Theresa. The economically successful nurse in private practice may be seen wearing designer clothes but not advertising as a nurse in the yellow pages. However, somewhere in these folds of silk, as long as this person identifies with the nursing profession, there still seems to beat the heart of a social activist who rises up to speak for the chronically ill, the poor, the elderly, abused women and children and the victims of crimes against society. Simultaneously then two images flash that must be termed "nurse." Will the real nurse please stand up!

It's provocative, but true that both images are accurate and reflect some movement of nursing. We promised in 1971 to watch more sunsets, eat more ice cream and fewer beans and to pick more daisies and take life less seriously. Nurses didn't do that as evidenced by more nurses becoming specialized practitioners and others getting baccalaureate and higher degrees. More, and hopefully, better higher education has certainly made nurses less content to be on the bottom of the totem pole earning less than less prepared people. Economically we command higher salaries than we did twelve years ago and some of us may be surprised to find that we do better than we ever expected in nursing *but*, and the 'but' is a big one compared to what? For instance the disparity ratio between what nurses get paid and what physicians get paid has widened from 1:2 ratio in 1935 to 1:10 in 1980.[3] The disparity ratio is wider than the mouths of Jaws I, II, and III.

Economics influence our image! What we charge in private practice and what we get paid in salaried positions is as it has always been a reflection of our collective self-worth. These past twelve years have seen nurses nationwide choose to collectively bargain when other negotiations around practice settings and economic worth have failed. Some have been successful and others less

[3] Kalisch, B. J., and P. A. Kalisch, Politics of Nursing, Philadelphia: J. B. Lippincott, 1982, p. 13.

so and nursing has had deep divisions within it as to how to attain economic status. There is no one outside of our profession to help us with this and much within to prevent it from happening. So back again to our image and how we can use it to project our worth to ourselves first and then to the public. On a Kraft sugar package is a definition of Advertising that reads, "He who has a thing to sell and goes and whispers in a well, is not so apt to get the dollars as he who climbs a tree and hollers."

The Kalisches describe, in magazine articles and in their book *The Advance of American Nursing*, nurses in the movies through the years, including the war years, where the image of nurse was that of a heroine who even achieved officer's rank[4] and was seen as a "cool resourceful and efficient worker,"[5] (though this was a relative rank until after World War II). In recent years, in both visual medias—television and movies—, nursing's image has in most cases fared poorly.[6] Millions of people who watch daytime television's General Hospital see actresses called nurses almost always behind a desk filing papers and answering telephone messages for passing doctors, as well as hiding behind charts or looking seductive. The award winning two years of the hour length "Nurse" that earned the actress, Michael Learned, an "Emmy" earned few accolades from our group or the nurses with whom we talked.

"Nurse" unlike "General Hospital" probably didn't hurt our image but it is doubtful that it helped. It was, however, in these days when hero men are present in ever increasing numbers on television, one of the few serious programs with a woman as a heroine who happens to be a nurse.

MASH, of course, has the one nurse, Hotlips Houlihan—Major Margaret Houlihan—that all of our group of nurses we surveyed liked best—a sensitive, sensual bright person who could hold her own in most situations, whose intelligence and knowledge and whose sometimes abrasive style and rank was most of the time a-okay. To quote the Kalisches—"During the first several seasons, Margaret (then mockingly call Hotlips), the short tempered, hypercritical head nurse, was one of the bad guys,"[7] now, she is fully integrated into the good guys camp. . . . Hotlips' manner is, and was, a better image in both TV and movies as opposed to the psychiatric nurses portrayed in both "One Flew Over the Cuckoo's Nest" and the comedy "High Anxiety." If there ever was a profession that needed a spin-off of a leading character, it's Major Margaret Houlihan that our 1.4 million strong registered nurses ought

---

[4] Aynes, E. A. From Nightingale to Eagle. Englewood Cliffs, New Jersey, 1973, Prentice-Hall, Inc., p. 38.

[5] Kalisch, P., and B. Kalisch, The Advance of American Nursing, Boston, 1978, Little, Brown and Company, pp. 29–30, p. 48, pp. 76–86.

[6] Kalisch, P., and B. Kalisch, Nurses on Prime-Time Television, American Journal of Nursing, 1982 pp. 264–270.

[7] *Ibid,* pp. 269–270.

to ask for. Imagine now that the TV war in Korea is about to be over if Major Houlihan comes out of the service, joins the Reserves, goes back to get her B.S., if she doesn't have one, and becomes a community health nurse. Margaret could also choose to work on a medical surgical floor or in the emergency room or intensive care unit. (She's certainly had the experience, but maybe she's had enough). She could get her M.S. in mental health and try to find a job in a mental health center or get her Ph.D. and maybe shake up the nursing education system. Wow—what a possibility. It will be interesting to see what does happen. Our guess is that she'll just go down the tubes. The nurse mother in "The World According to Garp," both the book and movie, is of interest as feminist and a nurse; the television programs such as CBS Reports—Nurse Where Are You?, the PBS programs on midwives, most of whom were nurses, have been noteworthy. These are mere drops in a big bucket when one considers we nurses represent the most women in any one professional group. It wouldn't hurt the 2 percent male members of our profession to have image building in the media for the profession. How about Hotlips marrying a male nurse?

The power of power

In 1983 it comes down to the issue of power again but for what end do we want power? The authors think the ends are these:

1) The power to influence the health care system for the benefit of the patient;
2) The power to influence the economic system for our own benefit;
3) The power-prestige of being recognized as a peer and colleague on the health care team, and
4) The power to advance our profession to the limits of knowledge in science and art.

We cannot have ambivalence, passivity, or indecisiveness if we are to attain such goals. In the 1971 book we used a quote on power from *Look* magazine to close the book. In 1983 we will refer you to and use some quotes from *MS Magazine*—December, 1982 issue on Women and Power. Our male colleagues should be liberated enough not to mind because in increasing the consciousness of the 98 percent female members of our profession we help the 2 percent male as well.

"The problem," says Margaret Henning, "is that the world works for men in power the way it is, and you must teach women to survive in that world 'as it is' . . . We must acquire the functional knowledge and the managerial skills which men already possess . . . But," she stresses, "this does not mean that you must renounce your vision of the world as you want it to be. Women with power do not have to act like men with power. They do not have to be co-opted."

. . . Is there a distinctively female style of power? Rosabeth Moss Kanter has found that women and men in senior management vary more as individuals than as representatives of their respective sexes. "Power wipes sex out," she asserts. But this does not mean that powerful women act "like men." Good managers seem to have the "human" relational skills associated with women and the "leadership" skills associated with men. They inspire confidence in their superiors and loyalty in their subordinates by getting things done. And they understand the value of "empowering" others.[8]

And to continue . . .

Women's progress, women's equality, are intimately connected to the issue of women's power. On the one hand, we have, at least for the next few years, buried the Equal Rights Amendment. A reactionary backlash threatens our hard-won freedoms. We are faced with an economy in which affirmative-action programs are being scrapped, women and minorities laid off, and conservative politics and attitudes gaining the high ground. The majority of women who work are filling traditional "women's jobs," where they are underpaid and discriminated against for promotion.

On the other hand, the majority of women do work outside the home, and expect to work for most of their lives. The old patterns of dependence are being changed by economic necessity, by the self-confidence that comes from action, and through the solidarity fostered by the Women's Movement. The number of women in management has more than doubled, and one in three MBA candidates is female. If women in the Senate, on the police force, anchoring the news, running the courts, the banks, the factories and the resources of this country are still a numerically insignificant elite—sometimes espousing elite politics—they are still of incalculable moral value to us. They are setting the precedents for the next generation, and they are creating a reality, a way to think about and perceive powerful women, where before we only had myths or caricatures. (Leathery old Ma Hawkins, riding roughshod over "the boys"; virginal Saint Joan with her haggard eyes and her inner voices; the Eve Arden-style boss lady, all tailoring and repartee—and secretly longing to doff her shoulder pads and "surrender."

---

[8] Thurman, J. All About Power—The Drives, The Hang-ups, The Joys, The Price. *Ms.*, December, 1982, p. 46.

Perhaps the greatest change wrought by feminism in the last decade—and perhaps the most radical change of this century—has been to establish women's presence in the "power" sphere as socially, politically, economically, and psychologically legitimate.[9]

In 1983, just as it was in 1971, this is what it is all about for the profession of nursing.

---

[9]Thurman, op. cit., p. 78.

Epilogue

K-K-Keystone

For those of you who may have purchased the first edition of Out of Uniform you might recall that we used the epilogue to share with our readers about us and how we wrote. We will do the same in this book.

The first edition was written in a rented cabin in Bailey, Colorado as we felt we could be more creative in an atmosphere away from the urban sprawl and in a mountainous setting. This edition has been written in a time shared condominium in Keystone, Colorado, in a mountain setting away from the urban sprawl. As far as we are concerned our creative juices flowed more easily there than in the cities where our primary jobs are. We had a little fun too.

In the preface we told you that our original Task Force had changed to a gang of three. Our gang of three was actually composed of a terrific twosome who did the writing in Keystone and a modern day Margaret Mead who after depositing her twenty-six page epistle took off to Australia. We managed to get the three of us together via overseas telephone and in spirit and then in the flesh in Denver in December. A snowstorm limited the direct contact we had so long anticipated to complete the book. Phone calls and reading chapters and finally a get-together at Stapleton Airport before Margaret Mead flew off again got the book done.

As was mentioned, our original Task Force had changed during the last twelve years. Two of the original members were deceased and each of us had suffered tragedies as well as survived triumphs. We had split geographically; one remained in Denver during the decade but traveled worldwide to exotic shores in her Mead-like garb with Pith helmet and field notepad. She also teaches in a doctoral program for psychosocial nursing and emerges weekly from the ivory tower to work as a staff nurse in an acute care psychiatric setting in a private hospital. One left Denver only to come back to re-establish her identity after a sojourn as an executive director of a State Nurses Association and as director of a day hospital program in a nursing home as well as an outpatient psychotherapist in a quasi mental health center in Massachusetts. Once back in Colorado she worked for a year with chronic patients in a community mental health center and then became a state nursing consultant supervisor with the Colorado Department of Health. She has been instrumental in the development of media presentations on the role of the community health nurse. CBS Sunday Morning News devoted a segment of one of its programs on the role of the nurse in rural public health through her efforts. The former director of a multi dimensional community mental health program in Denver is now settled in, hot tub and all, in Billings, Montana, where for the last decade of her life she has been the administrator and consultant of a mental health program for native Americans. She has been instrumental in the development of children's mental health services, started alcoholism services in her region and also served on and chaired the American Nurses' Association Psychiatric Nursing Certification Board. She has traveled the entire country either through job related activities or in ANA sponsored programs so has seen nurses all over. Her healthy life style from daily running to Haagen Dazs ice cream is of envy.

Over the last several years the three of us who authored this edition kept finding a fascinating phenomenon. This phenomenon was that whenever we presented a paper or were introduced to an audience and it was mentioned that we had been part of the Task Force that wrote *Out of Uniform and Into Trouble* the response was positive. Nurse strangers would come forth acting and obviously feeling like old friends with a pat or a hug and saying such things as ". . . the book became my Bible" or ". . . I made everyone of my students read it . . .they need to know the real world." One of us even had the "chilling" experience of being examined by a nurse who left our author sitting with nothing but those paper gowns that leave you bare in the back only to have the nurse return with the first edition of the book to be autographed. So, whenever we had a chance to see or talk to each other and since two of us now owned the copyright we discussed the possibility of publishing it. We tossed around publishing it ourselves as we felt unwilling to turn over our own creative and imaginative ideas to a publisher, but we also realized that we might never get done without the contractual commitments that a publisher would give us. Our faculty member, modern Margaret Mead, felt that the Charles B. Slack publishing company met our needs in terms of their forward thinking ideas and fresh alert public relations people and they were interested. After many negotiations and assurances that Slack would indeed meet our needs, contracts were signed and away we went to bring this book to you.

Twelve years ago we knew we had something different to give to our profession and people interested in our profession. The reviews then and the comments of people throughout the years validated that. We hope this new-old book is as provocative as the first and, as our median age now is forty-six, we'd just as soon have more immediate reaction to *this* book. Perhaps we need to write a book on nursing in general using this style. We welcome your response to our endeavors with the same hopes we had at the end of our first edition and with less fear and trembling.

Bibliography 1983

Aynes, E. From Nightingale to Eagle. Englewood Cliffs, N. J.: Prentice-Hall, Inc., 1973.

Colorado Division of Mental Health Report, 1981.

Colorado Mental Health Manpower: An empirical study. Western Interstate Commission for Higher Education, Boulder, Colorado, 1971.

Colorado Nurse's Association Resolution, House of Delegates Report, April, 1981.

Colorado Private Sector Mental Health Survey, 1980, Mental Health Association of Colorado, 1981.

Colorado Public Health Association Resolution Convention Report, June, 1981.

Job Description Health Care Technician 1–4, Denver Health and Hospital Career Service Authority, June 1, 1980.

Kalisch, P.A., and B. Kalisch. The Advance of American Nursing. Boston: Little, Brown and Company, 1978.

Kalisch, B., and P. Kalisch. Politics in Nursing. Philadelphia: J.B. Lippincott Co., 1982.

Kalisch, P., and B. Kalisch. Nurses on Prime-Time Television. American Journal of Nursing, February, 1982.

Osborne, D. Rich Doctors, Poor Nurses. Harper's, September, 1982.

NURSE Inc. A Case for Cooking. Denver, Colorado, 1980.

Schorr, T.M. Nursing Leaders, an Endangered Species. Editorial, American Journal of Nursing, February, 1982.

Thurman, J. All about Power—The Drives, The Hang-ups, The Joys, The Price . . . MS Magazine, December, 1982.

Vaughn, J. Educational Preparation for Nursing, 1981. Nursing and Health Care, Vol. 3, No. 8, 1982.

Western Interstate Commission for Higher Education, Newsletter, Winter, 1982.

Bibliography 1971

Albee, G. W.: No magic here, Contemporary Psychology, Vol. 10, Sept. 1965.

The Battle Over Nurses: Medical World News, McGraw-Hill, Inc., Nov. 21, 1969.

Bonn, E. M.: A therapeutic community in an open state hospital. Administrative-therapeutic links, Hospital and Community Psychiatry 20(9) Sept. 1969.

Brackbill, G. A.: Psychologists and nurses in the mental hospital, Journal of Psychiatric Nursing, Sept.-Oct. 1967.

Chance, E., and Arnold, J.: The effect of professional training, experience and preference for a theoretical system upon clinical care, description, Human Relations, Aug. 1960.

Christman, L.: Nurse-physician communication, Journal of the American Medical Association 194(5) Nov. 1, 1965.

Corwin, R. G., and Taves, M. J.: Nursing and other health professions. In Freeman, H. E., Levine, S., and Reeder, L. G., editors: Handbook of medical sociology, Englewood Cliffs, N.J., Prentice-Hall, 1963.

Dolan, J.: History of nursing, ed. 12, Philadelphia, 1968, W. B. Saunders Co.

Dorsett, C.: New directions in mental health facilities, The American Institute of Architects, Nov. 1964.

Freeman, H. E., and Gertner, R.S.: The changing posture of the mental health consortium, American Journal of Orthopsychiatry 39(1), Jan. 1969.

Gebbie, K. M., Deloughery, G., and Neuman, B. M.: Levels of utilization: nursing specialists in community mental health, Journal of Psychiatric Nursing, Vol. 8, No. 1, Jan.-Feb. 1970.

Glittenberg, J. A.: The role of the nurse in outpatient psychiatric clinics, The American Journal of Orthopsychiatry 39:1, July 1963.

Goffman, E.: Stigma: Notes on the management of a spoiled identity, Englewood Cliffs, N.J., 1965, Prentice-Hall, Inc.

Harrington, H., and Theis, E. C.: Institutional factors perceived by baccalaureate graduates as influencing their performance as staff nurses, Nursing Research, Vol. 17, No. 3, May-June 1968.

Hedges, F.: A brief history of the Colorado Psychiatric Technicians' Association. In Fuzessery, Z., editor: New frontiers in psychiatric technology, Second Annual Education Workshop of the Colorado Psychiatric Technicians' Association, Pueblo, Colorado, April 1969.

Hughes, E.: States—dilemmas and contradictions of states, In Coser, L.A., and others, editors: Sociological theory: a book of readings, N.Y., 1965, The Macmillan Co.

Joint Commission on Mental Health of Children: Crisis in child mental health; challenge for the 70's, New York, 1970, Harper & Row.

Jones, M.: The therapeutic community, New York, 1953, Basic Books, Inc., Publishers.

Jourard, S. M.: Speech presented at 3rd Annual Henrietta Loughran Seminar Series, Denver, Colorado, January 27, 1970.

Jourard, S. M.: Suicide—an invitation to die, American Journal of Nursing, Vol 70, No. 2, Feb. 1970.

Komisar, L.: The new feminism, Saturday Review, Feb. 21, 1970.

Krueger, C.: Do bad girls become good nurses, Transaction, July-Aug. 1968.

Lamb, R. H., Heath, D., and Downing, J. J. In Bowen, P., and others, editors: Handbook of community mental health practice, San Francisco, 1969, Jossey-Bass, Inc., Publishers.

Leifer, R.: In the name of mental health, New York, 1969, Science House, Inc.

Leonard, G. B.: The future of power, Look Magazine, Jan. 13, 1970.

Loeb, M. B.: Some dominant cultural themes in a psychiatric hospital. In Spitzer, S. P., and Denzin, N. K., editors: The mental patient; studies in the sociology of deviance, New York, 1968, McGraw-Hill Book Co.

Meyer, G. R.: The attitude of student nurses toward patient contact and their images of and preferences for four nursing specialties, Nursing Research, Vol. 7, Oct. 1958.

Miller, A. A., and others: Psychotherapy in psychiatric hospitals: a proposed model for psychiatrist-nurse-patient interaction, Archives of General Psychiatry, Vol. A, July 1963.

Nurses, Nursing and the A.N.A: The American Journal of Nursing **70**:4, April 1970.

Olesen, V. L., and Davis, F.: Baccalaureate students; images of nursing—a follow-up report, Nursing Research, Vol. 15, No. 2, Spring 1966.

Parsons, T.: On becoming a patient. In Folta, J. R., and Deck, E. S., editors: A sociological framework for patient care, New York, 1966, John Wiley & Sons.

Patterson, L.: Whose values? Colorado Psychiatric Technicians' Association, Feb. 1970.

Peter, L. J., and Hull, R.: The Peter principle—why things always go wrong. New York, 1969, William Morrow & Co., Inc.

Reres, M. E.: A survey of the nurse's role in psychiatric outpatient clinics in America: Community Mental Health Journal **5**:5, Oct. 1969.

Rogatz, P.: The health care system, Hospitals, Vol. 44, April 1970.

Rushing, W. A.: Social influence and social-psychological function of deference: a study of psychiatric nursing. In Skipper, J. K., and Leonard, R. C., editors: Social interaction and patient care, Philadelphia, 1965, J. B. Lippincott Co.

Sarosi, G. M.: A critical theory: the nurse as a fully human person, Nursing Forum, Vol. 7, No. 4, 1968.

Schiff, S. B.: A therapeutic community in an open state hospital. Administrative framework for social psychology, Hospital and Community Psychiatry, Vol. 20, No. 9, Sept. 1969.

Scott, W. G.: Human relations in management, Homewood, Ill., 1962, Richard D. Irwin, Inc.

Smith, L. M.: The system—barriers to quality nursing. In Folta, J. R., and Deck, E. S., editors: A sociological framework for patient care, New York, 1966, John Wiley & Sons, Inc.

Spindler, G. D.: Group values—traditional to emergent. In Carter, H. J., editor: Intellectual foundations of American education, New York, 1965, Pitman Publishing Corp.

Stachyra, M.: Nurses, psychotherapy, and the law, Perspectives in Psychiatric Care, Vol. 7, Nov. 5, 1969.

Stein, L. I.: The doctor-nurse game, Archives of General Psychiatry, Vol. 16, June 1967.

Stokes, G. A., Williams, F. S., Davidites, R. M., Bulbulyan, A., and Ullman, M.: The roles of psychiatric nurses in community mental health practice: a giant step, New York, 1969, Faculty Press, Inc.

Torrey, F. E.: The case for the indigenous therapist, Archives of General Psychiatry, Vol. 20, March 1969.

Von Ende, Z.: Panel of women lashes alleged injustices in 'men's world', The Denver Post, Friday, May 1, 1970, Denver, Colo.

Yolles, S. F.: The role of the psychologist in comprehensive community health center, American Psychologist, Jan. 1966.

Zahourek, R., and Tower, M.: Community mental health nurses question care, cure and coordination, Conference on Nursing in Community Mental Health Centers of the American Nurses' Association, New York, February 26, 1970, American Journal of Nursing, Vol 70, No. 5, May 1970.

Appendix

Questions of the Task Force of the Psychiatric-Mental Health Group (to determine the role of the nurse in the comprehensive community mental health center)

1. Given the five basic components:
   (a) Inpatient
   (b) Outpatient (aftercare)
   (c) Partial hospitalization
   (d) Consultation, research, education
   (e) Emergency service
   How do you see the role of the nurse in these areas?

2. What would you consider the basic preparation for the nurse in the comprehensive community health center, in the areas cited in the previous question? Would you consider additional preparation necessary?

3. What would be some of your ideas for ways we might implement whatever results we come up with in planning for Colorado?

INDEX